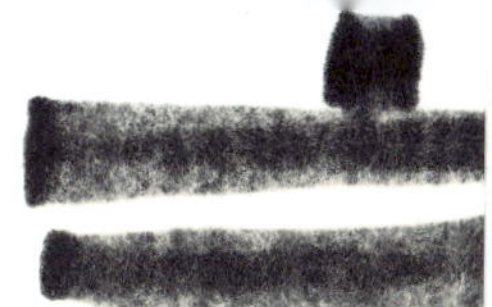

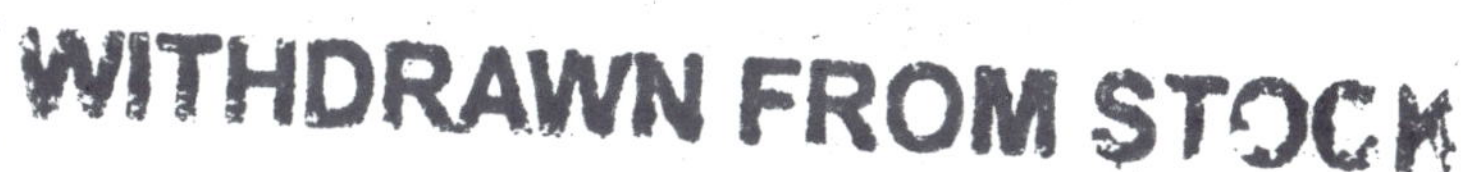

THE RHESUS FACTOR AND DISEASE PREVENTION

The transcript of a Witness Seminar held by the Wellcome Trust Centre for the History of Medicine at UCL, London, on 3 June 2003

Edited by D T Zallen, D A Christie and E M Tansey

Volume 22 2004

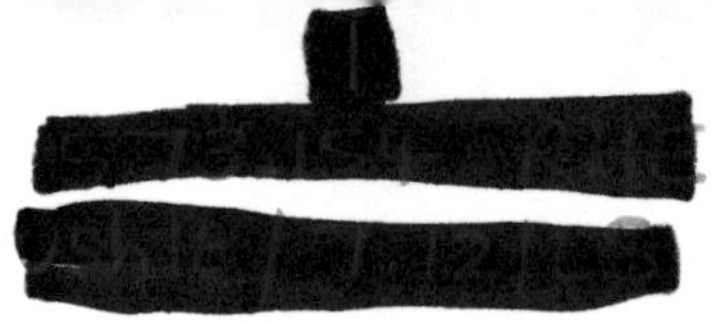

First published by the Wellcome Trust Centre
for the History of Medicine at UCL, 2004

The Wellcome Trust Centre for the History of Medicine
at University College London is funded by the Wellcome Trust,
which is a registered charity, no. 210183.

ISBN 0 85484 099 0

Histmed logo images courtesy Wellcome Library, London.

Design and production: Julie Wood at Shift Key Design 020 7241 3704

**For details of other volumes in the series, visit
www.ucl.ac.uk/histmed/witnesses.html**

Technology Transfer in Britain: The case of monoclonal antibodies; Self and Non-Self: A history of autoimmunity; Endogenous Opiates; The Committee on Safety of Drugs • Making the Human Body Transparent: The impact of NMR and MRI; Research in General Practice; Drugs in Psychiatric Practice; The MRC Common Cold Unit • Early Heart Transplant Surgery in the UK • Haemophilia: Recent history of clinical management • Looking at the Unborn: Historical aspects of obstetric ultrasound • Post Penicillin Antibiotics: From acceptance to resistance? • Clinical Research in Britain, 1950–1980 • Intestinal Absorption • Origins of Neonatal Intensive Care in the UK • British Contributions to Medical Research and Education in Africa after the Second World War • Childhood Asthma and Beyond • Maternal Care • Population-based Research in South Wales: The MRC Pneumoconiosis Research Unit and the MRC Epidemiology Unit • Peptic Ulcer: Rise and fall • Leukaemia • The MRC Applied Psychology Unit • Genetic Testing • Foot and Mouth Disease: The 1967 outbreak and its aftermath • Environmental Toxicology: The legacy of *Silent Spring* • Cystic Fibrosis

CONTENTS

ILLUSTRATIONS AND CREDITS

WITNESS SEMINARS: MEETINGS AND PUBLICATIONS[1]

In 1990 the Wellcome Trust created a History of Twentieth Century Medicine Group, as part of the Academic Unit of the Wellcome Institute for the History of Medicine, to bring together clinicians, scientists, historians and others interested in contemporary medical history. Among a number of other initiatives the format of Witness Seminars, used by the Institute of Contemporary British History to address issues of recent political history, was adopted, to promote interaction between these different groups, to emphasize the potential benefits of working jointly, and to encourage the creation and deposit of archival sources for present and future use. In June 1999 the Governors of the Wellcome Trust decided that it would be appropriate for the Academic Unit to enjoy a more formal academic affiliation and turned the Unit into the Wellcome Trust Centre for the History of Medicine at University College London from 1 October 2000. The Wellcome Trust continues to fund the Witness Seminar programme via its support for the Centre.

The Witness Seminar is a particularly specialized form of oral history, where several people associated with a particular set of circumstances or events are invited to come together to discuss, debate, and agree or disagree about their memories. To date, the History of Twentieth Century Medicine Group has held nearly 40 such meetings, most of which have been published, as listed on pages xi–xviii.

Subjects are usually proposed by, or through, members of the Programme Committee of the Group, and once an appropriate topic has been agreed, suitable participants are identified and invited. This inevitably leads to further contacts, and more suggestions of people to invite. As the organization of the meeting progresses, a flexible outline plan for the meeting is devised, usually with assistance from the meeting's chairman, and some participants are invited to 'set the ball rolling' on particular themes, by speaking for a short period to initiate and stimulate further discussion.

Each meeting is fully recorded, the tapes are transcribed and the unedited transcript is immediately sent to every participant. Each is asked to check his or her own contributions and to provide brief biographical details. The editors

[1] The following text also appears in the 'Introduction' to recent volumes of *Wellcome Witnesses to Twentieth Century Medicine* published by the Wellcome Trust and the Wellcome Trust Centre for the History of Medicine at University College London.

turn the transcript into readable text, and participants' minor corrections and comments are incorporated into that text, while biographical and bibliographical details are added as footnotes, as are more substantial comments and additional material provided by participants. The final scripts are then sent to every contributor, accompanied by forms assigning copyright to the Wellcome Trust. Copies of all additional correspondence received during the editorial process are deposited with the records of each meeting in Archives and Manuscripts, Wellcome Library, London.

As with all our meetings, we hope that even if the precise details of some of the technical sections are not clear to the non-specialist, the sense and significance of the events will be understandable. Our aim is for the volumes that emerge from these meetings to inform those with a general interest in the history of modern medicine and medical science; to provide historians with new insights, fresh material for study, and further themes for research; and to emphasize to the participants that events of the recent past, of their own working lives, are of proper and necessary concern to historians.

ACKNOWLEDGEMENTS

'The Rhesus Factor and Disease Prevention' was suggested as a suitable topic for a Witness Seminar by Professor Doris Zallen, who provided many of the names of individuals to be invited, and helped decide on the topics to be discussed. We are particularly grateful to her for writing the Introduction to these published proceedings. We are equally grateful to Professor Sir David Weatherall for his excellent chairing of the occasion. Additional thanks are due to Professor Doris Zallen and Professor John Woodrow for assistance. Dr Sheila Duncan, Dr Belinda Kumpel, Professor Patrick Mollison, Professor Charles Rodeck, Dr Derrick Tovey and Professor John Walker-Smith provided the photographs.

As with all our meetings, we depend a great deal on our colleagues at the Wellcome Trust to ensure their smooth running: the Audiovisual Department, the Medical Photographic Library and Mrs Tracy Tillotson of the Wellcome Library; Ms Julie Wood, who has supervised the design and production of this volume; our indexer, Ms Liza Furnival, and our readers, Ms Kathryn Merritt, Mr Richard Barnett and Mr Simon Reynolds. Mrs Jaqui Carter is our transcriber, and Mrs Wendy Kutner and Mrs Lois Reynolds assist us in running the meetings. Finally we thank the Wellcome Trust for supporting this programme.

Tilli Tansey

Daphne Christie

Wellcome Trust Centre for the History of Medicine at UCL

HISTORY OF TWENTIETH CENTURY MEDICINE WITNESS SEMINARS, 1993–2005

1993 **Monoclonal antibodies**
Organizers: Dr E M Tansey and Dr Peter Catterall

1994 **The early history of renal transplantation**
Organizer: Dr Stephen Lock

Pneumoconiosis of coal workers
Organizer: Dr E M Tansey

1995 **Self and non-self: A history of autoimmunity**
Organizers: Sir Christopher Booth and Dr E M Tansey

Ashes to ashes: The history of smoking and health
Organizers: Dr Stephen Lock and Dr E M Tansey

Oral contraceptives
Organizers: Dr Lara Marks and Dr E M Tansey

Endogenous opiates
Organizer: Dr E M Tansey

1996 **Committee on Safety of Drugs**
Organizers: Dr Stephen Lock and Dr E M Tansey

Making the body more transparent: The impact of nuclear magnetic resonance and magnetic resonance imaging
Organizer: Sir Christopher Booth

1997 **Research in General Practice**
Organizers: Dr Ian Tait and Dr E M Tansey

Drugs in psychiatric practice
Organizers: Dr David Healy and Dr E M Tansey

The MRC Common Cold Unit
Organizers: Dr David Tyrrell and Dr E M Tansey

The first heart transplant in the UK
Organizer: Professor Tom Treasure

1998 **Haemophilia: Recent history of clinical management**
Organizers: Professor Christine Lee and Dr E M Tansey

Obstetric ultrasound: Historical perspectives
Organizers: Dr Malcolm Nicolson, Mr John Fleming and Dr E M Tansey

Post penicillin antibiotics
Organizers: Dr Robert Bud and Dr E M Tansey

Clinical research in Britain, 1950–1980
Organizers: Dr David Gordon and Dr E M Tansey

1999 **Intestinal absorption**
Organizers: Sir Christopher Booth and Dr E M Tansey

The MRC Epidemiology Unit (South Wales)
Organizers: Dr Andy Ness and Dr E M Tansey

Neonatal intensive care
Organizers: Professor Osmund Reynolds and Dr E M Tansey

British contributions to medicine in Africa after the Second World War
Organizers: Dr Mary Dobson, Dr Maureen Malowany, Dr Gordon Cook and Dr E M Tansey

2000 **Childhood asthma, and beyond**
Organizers: Dr Chris O'Callaghan and Dr Daphne Christie

Peptic ulcer: Rise and fall
Organizers: Sir Christopher Booth, Professor Roy Pounder and Dr E M Tansey

Maternal care
Organizers: Dr Irvine Loudon and Dr Daphne Christie

2001 **Leukaemia**
Organizers: Professor Sir David Weatherall, Professor John Goldman, Sir Christopher Booth and Dr Daphne Christie

The MRC Applied Psychology Unit
Organizers: Dr Geoff Bunn and Dr Daphne Christie

Genetic testing
Organizers: Professor Doris Zallen and Dr Daphne Christie

Foot and mouth disease: the 1967 outbreak and its aftermath
Organizers: Dr Abigail Woods, Dr Daphne Christie and Dr David Aickin

2002 **Environmental toxicology: The legacy of *Silent Spring***
Organizers: Dr Robert Flanagan and Dr Daphne Christie

Cystic fibrosis
Organizers: Dr James Littlewood and Dr Daphne Christie

Innovation in pain management
Organizers: Professor David Clark and Dr Daphne Christie

2003 **Thrombolysis**
Organizers: Mr Robert Arnott and Dr Daphne Christie

Beyond the asylum: Anti-psychiatry and care in the community
Organizers: Dr Mark Jackson and Dr Daphne Christie

The Rhesus factor and disease prevention
Organizers: Professor Doris Zallen and Dr Daphne Christie

Platelets in thrombosis and other disorders
Organizers: Professor Gustav Born and Dr Daphne Christie

2004 **Short course chemotherapy for tuberculosis**
Organizers: Dr Owen McCarthy and Dr Daphne Christie

Prenatal corticosteroids for reducing morbidity and mortality associated with preterm birth
Organizers: Sir Iain Chalmers and Dr Daphne Christie

Public health in the 1980s and 1990s: Decline and rise?
Organizers: Professor Virginia Berridge, Dr Niki Ellis and Dr Daphne Christie

2005 **The history of cholesterol, atherosclerosis and coronary disease**
Organizers: Professor Michael Oliver and Dr Daphne Christie

Development of physics applied to medicine
Organizers: Professor John Clifton and Dr Daphne Christie

PUBLISHED MEETINGS

"...Few books are so intellectually stimulating or uplifting".
Journal of the Royal Society of Medicine (1999) **92:** 206–8,
review of vols 1 and 2

"...This is oral history at its best...all the volumes make compulsive reading...they are, primarily, important historical records".
British Medical Journal (2002) **325**: 1119, review of the series

Technology transfer in Britain: The case of monoclonal antibodies
Self and non-self: A history of autoimmunity
Endogenous opiates
The Committee on Safety of Drugs
In: Tansey E M, Catterall P P, Christie D A, Willhoft S V, Reynolds L A. (eds) (1997) *Wellcome Witnesses to Twentieth Century Medicine.* Volume 1. London: The Wellcome Trust, 135pp. ISBN 1 869835 79 4

Making the human body transparent: The impact of NMR and MRI
Research in General Practice
Drugs in psychiatric practice
The MRC Common Cold Unit
In: Tansey E M, Christie D A, Reynolds L A. (eds) (1998) *Wellcome Witnesses to Twentieth Century Medicine.* Volume 2. London: The Wellcome Trust, 282pp. ISBN 1 869835 39 5

Early heart transplant surgery in the UK
In: Tansey E M, Reynolds L A. (eds) (1999) *Wellcome Witnesses to Twentieth Century Medicine.* Volume 3. London: The Wellcome Trust, 72pp. ISBN 1 841290 07 6

Haemophilia: Recent history of clinical management
In: Tansey E M, Christie D A. (eds) (1999) *Wellcome Witnesses to Twentieth Century Medicine.* Volume 4. London: The Wellcome Trust, 90pp. ISBN 1 841290 08 4

Looking at the unborn: Historical aspects of obstetric ultrasound
In: Tansey E M, Christie D A. (eds) (2000) *Wellcome Witnesses to Twentieth*

Century Medicine. Volume 5. London: The Wellcome Trust, 80pp.
ISBN 1 841290 11 4

Post penicillin antibiotics: From acceptance to resistance?
In: Tansey E M, Reynolds L A. (eds) (2000) *Wellcome Witnesses to Twentieth Century Medicine*. Volume 6. London: The Wellcome Trust, 71pp.
ISBN 1 841290 12 2

Clinical research in Britain, 1950–1980
In: Reynolds L A, Tansey E M. (eds) (2000) *Wellcome Witnesses to Twentieth Century Medicine*. Volume 7. London: The Wellcome Trust, 74pp.
ISBN 1 841290 16 5

Intestinal absorption
In: Christie D A, Tansey E M. (eds) (2000) *Wellcome Witnesses to Twentieth Century Medicine*. Volume 8. London: The Wellcome Trust, 81pp.
ISBN 1 841290 17 3

Neonatal intensive care
In: Christie D A, Tansey E M. (eds) (2001) *Wellcome Witnesses to Twentieth Century Medicine*. Volume 9. London: The Wellcome Trust Centre for the History of Medicine at UCL, 84pp. ISBN 0 854840 76 1

British contributions to medical research and education in Africa after the Second World War
In: Reynolds L A, Tansey E M. (eds) (2001) *Wellcome Witnesses to Twentieth Century Medicine*. Volume 10. London: The Wellcome Trust Centre for the History of Medicine at UCL, 93pp. ISBN 0 854840 77 X

Childhood asthma and beyond
In: Reynolds L A, Tansey E M. (eds) (2001) *Wellcome Witnesses to Twentieth Century Medicine*. Volume 11. London: The Wellcome Trust Centre for the History of Medicine at UCL, 74pp. ISBN 0 854840 78 8

Maternal care
In: Christie D A, Tansey E M. (eds) (2001) *Wellcome Witnesses to Twentieth Century Medicine*. Volume 12. London: The Wellcome Trust Centre for the History of Medicine at UCL, 88pp. ISBN 0 854840 79 6

Population-based research in south Wales: The MRC Pneumoconiosis Research Unit and the MRC Epidemiology Unit
In: Ness A R, Reynolds L A, Tansey E M. (eds) (2002) *Wellcome Witnesses to Twentieth Century Medicine.* Volume 13. London: The Wellcome Trust Centre for the History of Medicine at UCL, 74pp. ISBN 0 854840 81 8

Peptic ulcer: Rise and fall
In: Christie D A, Tansey E M. (eds) (2002) *Wellcome Witnesses to Twentieth Century Medicine.* Volume 14. London: The Wellcome Trust Centre for the History of Medicine at UCL, 143pp. ISBN 0 854840 84 2

Leukaemia
In: Christie D A, Tansey E M. (eds) (2003) *Wellcome Witnesses to Twentieth Century Medicine.* Volume 15. London: The Wellcome Trust Centre for the History of Medicine at UCL, 86pp. ISBN 0 85484 087 7

The MRC Applied Psychology Unit
In: Reynolds L A, Tansey E M. (eds) (2003) *Wellcome Witnesses to Twentieth Century Medicine.* Volume 16. London: The Wellcome Trust Centre for the History of Medicine at UCL, 94pp. ISBN 0 85484 088 5

Genetic testing
In: Christie D A, Tansey E M. (eds) (2003) *Wellcome Witnesses to Twentieth Century Medicine.* Volume 17. London: The Wellcome Trust Centre for the History of Medicine at UCL, 130pp. ISBN 0 85484 094 X

Foot and mouth disease: The 1967 outbreak and its aftermath
In: Reynolds L A, Tansey E M. (eds) (2003) *Wellcome Witnesses to Twentieth Century Medicine.* Volume 18. London: The Wellcome Trust Centre for the History of Medicine at UCL, 114pp. ISBN 0 85484 096 6

Environmental toxicology: The legacy of *Silent Spring*
In: Christie D A, Tansey E M. (eds) (2004) *Wellcome Witnesses to Twentieth Century Medicine.* Volume 19. London: The Wellcome Trust Centre for the History of Medicine at UCL, 132pp. ISBN 0 85484 091 5

Cystic fibrosis
In: Christie D A, Tansey E M. (eds) (2004) *Wellcome Witnesses to Twentieth Century Medicine.* Volume 20. London: The Wellcome Trust Centre for the History of Medicine at UCL, 120pp. ISBN 0 85484 086 9

Innovation in pain management
In: Reynolds L A, Tansey E M. (eds) (2004) *Wellcome Witnesses to Twentieth Century Medicine.* Volume 21. London: The Wellcome Trust Centre for the History of Medicine at UCL, 125pp. ISBN 0 85484 097 4

The Rhesus factor and disease prevention
In: Zallen D T, Christie D A, Tansey E M. (eds) (2004) *Wellcome Witnesses to Twentieth Century Medicine.* Volume 22. London: The Wellcome Trust Centre for the History of Medicine at UCL, 98pp, this volume. ISBN 0 85484 099 0

Platelets in thrombosis and other disorders
In: Reynolds L A, Tansey E M. (eds) (2005) *Wellcome Witnesses to Twentieth Century Medicine.* Volume 23. London: The Wellcome Trust Centre for the History of Medicine at UCL, in press.

Short course chemotherapy for tuberculosis
In: Christie D A, Tansey E M. (eds) (2005) *Wellcome Witnesses to Twentieth Century Medicine.* Volume 24. London: The Wellcome Trust Centre for the History of Medicine at UCL, in press.

Volumes 1–12 cost £5 plus postage, with volumes 13–20 at £10 each. Orders of four or more volumes receive a 20 per cent discount. All 20 published volumes in the series are available at the special price of £115 plus postage. To order a copy contact t.tillotson@wellcome.ac.uk or by phone: +44 (0)20 7611 8486; or fax: +44 (0)20 7611 8703.

Volumes 21–22 are available at www.ucl.ac.uk/histmed/witnesses.html
A paperback copy can be ordered from www.amazon.co.uk

Other publications

Technology transfer in Britain: The case of monoclonal antibodies
In: Tansey E M, Catterall P P. (1993) *Contemporary Record* **9**: 409–44.

Monoclonal antibodies: A witness seminar on contemporary medical history
In: Tansey E M, Catterall P P. (1994) *Medical History* **38**: 322–7.

Chronic pulmonary disease in South Wales coalmines: An eye-witness account of the MRC surveys (1937–42)
In: P D'Arcy Hart, edited and annotated by E M Tansey. (1998) *Social History of Medicine* 11: 459–68.

Ashes to Ashes – The history of smoking and health
In: Lock S P, Reynolds L A, Tansey E M. (eds) (1998) Amsterdam: Rodopi BV, 228pp. ISBN 90420 0396 0 (Hfl 125) (hardback). Reprinted 2003.

Witnessing medical history. An interview with Dr Rosemary Biggs
Professor Christine Lee and Dr Charles Rizza (interviewers). (1998) *Haemophilia* 4: 769–77.

Members of the Programme Committee of the History of Twentieth Century Medicine Group

The Group's activities are overseen by the Programme Committee, which includes professional historians of medicine, practising scientists and clinicians. The Programme Committee during 2003–04 comprised:

Dr Tilli Tansey – Historian of Modern Medical Science, Wellcome Trust Centre at UCL, and Chair

Sir Christopher Booth – Wellcome Trust Centre at UCL, former Director, Clinical Research Centre, Northwick Park Hospital, London

Dr Robert Bud – Head of Life and Environmental Sciences, Science Museum, London

Dr Daphne Christie – Senior Research Assistant, Wellcome Trust Centre at UCL, and Organizing Secretary

Professor Hal Cook – Director, Wellcome Trust Centre at UCL

Professor Mark Jackson – Centre for Medical History, Exeter

Professor Ian McDonald – Harveian Librarian, Royal College of Physicians, London

INTRODUCTION

All too often, especially in popular accounts of medical history, significant medical advances seem to arrive effortlessly as if they were the obvious and inevitable next steps in a research process that had a clear fix on exactly how to get to the desired goal. Serious historical scholarship has revealed that, most often, this is definitely not the case. Dogged determination at the lab bench is affected by chance occurrences, setbacks, charismatic or conflicting personalities, and dozens of other factors which intervene and interconnect to create a complex dynamic as the research proceeds.

On 3 June 2003, a Wellcome Witness Seminar was convened to examine what certainly qualifies as one of the major medical advances of the twentieth century: the prevention of rhesus haemolytic disease – or erythroblastosis fetalis – in newborns. This disease can arise when there is an immunological clash between Rh-negative mothers and their Rh-positive fetuses. When such a clash occurs, it exacts a terrible toll. Over a period of only about 30 years, from roughly the 1940s to the 1970s, the basis of this life-threatening disorder was understood, treatments were perfected, and a highly successful means of prevention was developed and validated. Despite our familiarity with the general outline of this story, most of the details – the back story as it were – are not known. This Witness Seminar was organized to fill in the knowledge gaps and gain a clearer understanding of the way this significant achievement in medical science came about.

The transcript that follows is the complete record of the discussions at this Witness Seminar. It covers the first experiments with Rh typing, the exchange-transfusion and intrauterine-transfusion procedures developed by clinicians to treat affected newborns and fetuses, and the research efforts that ultimately produced a prevention in at-risk families.

The 'Rhesus Factor and Disease Prevention' Witness Seminar was also the occasion for laying to rest a controversy that had arisen among medical historians and science writers as they tried to understand the history of rhesus disease prevention. The lingering controversy involved the question: Who was the first person to suggest that anti-Rh antibody could be used to remove Rh-positive cells and prevent the sensitization of the Rh-negative mothers? Was it Ronald Finn, the physician/researcher who presented the idea at a meeting of the Liverpool Medical Institution? Or was it, as Cyril Clarke maintained, Clarke's wife and research assistant, Féo, who woke him one night saying,

'Give them (the Rh-negative mothers) anti-Rh' (page 40)[1] Even Philip Sheppard, Clarke's close colleague, was uncertain. In an interview (*c.* 1968) captured on audiotape and available at the John Innes Centre Archives,[2] he said only that it was Clarke who first mentioned the idea to him. At this Witness Seminar, Professor Ronald Finn offered an answer that appears to resolve the controversy (page 40 and note 93a).

In addition, the participants were able to bring the history up to date, showing how it influenced the development of the new fields of neonatal and fetal medicine, and identifying areas of the rhesus story that still pose challenges both in the laboratory and in the clinic.

There is much that we can learn from the discussions and each reader will surely come away better informed, albeit in different ways. There are, however, a few elements that we would like to highlight here – elements not usually recognized in the popular accounts – that not only contributed to the successful conclusion of this episode in medical history but that may also hold some lessons for investigators and funding agencies working in today's research environment:

- Although individuals around the world were working hard to improve the condition of the newborns and reduce the suffering of their families, there does not appear to have been a race in which various people or groups vied to become the victor. Instead, one hallmark of this far-flung research community was the spirit of cooperation that extended to the sharing of ideas, reagents, data, and experience as people worked to provide better modes of treatment and to achieve a means of prevention.
- Another feature that emerged in the discussions was the number of *collaborations* that arose, particularly those in which the collaborators had strikingly different training, areas of expertise, or worked in different types of institutional settings. The most prominent example is the collaboration that arose between Cyril Clarke (1907–2000), a physician in Liverpool, and Philip Sheppard (1921–76), an ecological geneticist working at Oxford. This partnership, initiated by their mutual interest in butterflies, soon involved joint work on projects in an area that was new to both of them: medical genetics. Ultimately, they extended their research agenda to include rhesus

---

[1] Clarke (1968).

[2] A very brief account of the prevention of Rh haemolytic disease is given in a recording of Professor Philip Sheppard, 18 March 1968, available in the Genetics Society Archive (1968; SID I, 1–180), John Innes Centre Archives, Norwich.

haemolytic disease. There were a number of other collaborations as well – such as with the Blood Transfusion Service, the medical genetics laboratory (under the direction of Victor McKusick) at Johns Hopkins University in Maryland (USA), researchers at the Ortho Pharmaceutical Corporation in New Jersey (USA), and with personnel in an USA penitentiary – that allowed novel ideas to be raised, explored, and tested (page 32).

- Many of the leading researchers could best be described as '*amateurs*' (pages 35, 38). They were physicians in Liverpool who cared for their patients during the day and then dealt with medical research projects – usually in the evening – after their clinical duties had concluded. At the beginning of their involvement in this research area, they had neither laboratory experience nor familiarity with many of the basic concepts. Nonetheless, they succeeded in putting forth and subjecting to experimental test the two-part 'Liverpool hypothesis': that transfer of Rh-positive cells into Rh-negative mothers typically occurred at birth, not throughout pregnancy, and that the rapid removal of those fetal cells from maternal blood with anti-Rh (anti-D) antibody could prevent sensitization.
- The research surrounding treatment and prevention was accomplished with *modest funding* (page 45). In the present-day environment of big science and big budgets, it seems surprising how limited was the funding for this research. When substantial amounts of external support did come, in the form of a major Nuffield Foundation grant to the Liverpool group, it was only after the major part of the testing of the Liverpool hypothesis had already been accomplished. This Nuffield support allowed the establishment of a medical genetics research facility at the University of Liverpool which went on to grow in size and make key contributions in several different areas of medical genetics in the years that followed. Sadly, the departure of some of the original researchers left that unit vulnerable and, despite its illustrious history, it no longer exists.
- The clinicians and researchers were fortunate in the timely arrival of *new technologies* – such as flexible catheters which greatly simplified the process of blood transfusions, the Kleihauer technique which was a crucial tool for measuring the presence of fetal cells in maternal blood, and the quantitative measure of anti-D antibody which permitted standardized anti-D delivery – and rapidly pressed them into service (pages 15, 18–19, 30–31, 43).

We are deeply grateful to all the participants in this Witness Seminar for their generosity in sharing their experiences. Decades later, we are still able to draw inspiration and guidance from these dedicated individuals.

Doris T Zallen

Virginia Polytechnic Institute and State University, Blacksburg, Virginia (USA)

THE RHESUS FACTOR AND DISEASE PREVENTION

The transcript of a Witness Seminar held by the Wellcome Trust Centre for the History of Medicine at UCL, London, on 3 June 2003

Edited by D T Zallen, D A Christie and E M Tansey

THE RHESUS FACTOR AND DISEASE PREVENTION

Participants

Professor David Anstee
Professor Neil Avent
Dr Derek Bangham
Dr Barry Benster
Dr Frank Boulton
Professor Robin Coombs
Dr Beryl Corner
Dr Mahes de Silva
Dr Sheila Duncan
Professor Ronald Finn*
Professor Ian Franklin
Professor Peter Harper
Dr Nevin Hughes-Jones
Dr Peter Hunter
Dr Belinda Kumpel
Mr Ian MacKenzie
Dr Edwin Massey
Professor Patrick Mollison
Dr Archie Norman
Mr Elliot Philipp
Dr Angela Robinson
Professor Charles Rodeck
Professor James Scott
Dr John Silver
Dr Jean Smellie
Dr Patricia Tippett
Dr Derrick Tovey
Professor Timos Valaes
Mr Humphry Ward
Professor Sir David Weatherall (Chair)
Professor Charles Whitfield
Professor John Woodrow
Professor Doris Zallen

Among those attending the meeting: Dr Joseph Angel, Dr Elizabeth Caffrey, Dr Anne Coombs, Dr Helen Dodsworth, Dr Christopher Everett, Professor Christine Gosden, Mr Luke Matthews, Professor Ursula Mittwoch, Professor Colin Normand, Professor Naomi Pfeffer, Dr Fiona Regan, Ms Freda Roberts, Dr Shona Towers, Professor Stan Urbaniak, Dr Anthony Wilkes, Professor Maureen Young

Apologies include: Professor Sir Walter Bodmer, Mrs M C Cooper, Dr Pamela Davies, Dr Ian Fraser, Professor John Davis, Professor Peter Dunn, Dr Ruth Hussey, Dr Richard McConnell†, Professor Tom Oppé, Dr David Rushton, Dr Betty Tucker, Dr David Tyrrell, Dr Bryan Walker, Professor Jonathan Wigglesworth

* Died 21 May 2004

† Died 21 October 2003

Professor Sir David Weatherall: We are going to go through the history of the development of the rhesus factor story and before we start I would like to ask Doris Zallen to begin with a historical introduction.

Professor Doris Zallen: I have been asked to give some historical context and raise some questions, and I will try to do all of that. When it comes to sorting out the history of a medical advance, it is always hard to know where to begin. But certainly a major historical landmark anchoring today's discussion would have to be the work of Karl Landsteiner in 1900, for which he won the Nobel Prize in 1930.[1] Landsteiner discovered the existence of the ABO blood groups, the cell surface substances produced by genes that endow individuals with their individual blood types: A, B, O and AB.[2] Landsteiner's scientific finding was pressed into service. Clinically, of course, it resulted in safer blood transfusions in humans. Scientifically, it fuelled research efforts to find other such blood group systems. Initially, very few studies of the blood group factors took place in Britain. It wasn't until the 1930s – when J B S Haldane began to use blood types as human traits in his population genetic studies and when R A Fisher took over the Galton Chair at UCL and set up a laboratory that focused on blood group research – that blood groups became an area of active research in the UK.[3]

One prominent outcome of research in the USA, and a crucial historical landmark for us today, was the discovery of the Rh factor. Credit for this discovery still remains the subject of debate. It formed the basis of a lifelong feud between the two protagonists, Philip Levine and Alexander Wiener. Both claimed to have found the Rh factor in 1937, although their actual publications came several years later.[4] Wiener said that he and Landsteiner discovered the Rh factor in humans while they were looking for antisera to as yet undetected blood group factors, and they were doing this by injecting rhesus monkey blood into rabbits and guinea-pigs. They named the new antigen, thus revealed, as the rhesus, or Rh antigen. When the antiserum to Rh was tested against human blood, they found that 85 per cent of their samples were Rh positive, 15 per cent were Rh negative. They delayed publication, they claimed, to improve the process of production of the anti-rhesus serum. Their

---

[1] Landsteiner (1900, 1901). See also Owen (2000).

[2] Landsteiner (1903); Rous (1947). See also Diamond (1980b).

[3] Bodmer (1992).

[4] Levine and Stetson (1939); Landsteiner and Wiener (1940); See also Wiener (1954, 1969); Levine (1984).

work was not published until 1940, three years after their initial studies, when it became clear that it could explain unexpected haemolytic reactions that arose during blood transfusions between otherwise ABO-identical individuals.

For his part, Levine thought he had priority. In 1937 he had found a previously unknown antiserum in a woman who had given birth to a stillborn infant. This antiserum reacted with the father's red blood cells, but not the mother's. The same antiserum also reacted with 80 per cent of other blood samples with which it was tested. Levine's publication on this case, co-authored with Rufus Stetson, didn't appear until 1939, two years later.[5] Why the delay? It's not clear, but there may have been serious disputes about authorship that arose within the group itself. What isn't disputed is that Wiener gave the new factor its name, Rh, and that Levine explained its role in the disease affecting the family whose blood he had studied in 1937.

The particular disease, erythroblastosis fetalis, was one that afflicted many newborns, about one in 200, and appeared again and again in the same families. Haemolytic diseases of the newborn had been known and reported in the medical literature. The first such report describing one of its features, hydrops fetalis, appeared in 400 BC,[6] but little was known of the cause. Levine had the answer. Rh antibody was formed in an Rh-negative woman when she was exposed to blood from her fetus, blood that contained the Rh factor. In this circumstance, the Rh antibody produced by the mother could cross the placenta and attack Rh-positive fetal cells, often with tragic results. What was this Rh factor? What were its properties? How was it inherited? Was there any way to treat the disease? Was there any way to prevent it? Different groups on both sides of the Atlantic focused their attention on these issues.

Today's Witness Seminar will bring us to the heart of the Rh factor story. Among the things we will be trying to discover are not only what happened and when – not only the timeline – but why it happened and how. How did Rh factor research take hold in a country where blood group research had been neglected for such a long time? How was it possible for a group of physicians at Liverpool to play such a significant role? This is a group that Cyril Clarke called 'amateurs'.[7] They were physicians who spent most of their time dealing with clinical duties. They weren't paediatricians, or obstetricians; they had

---

[5] See note 4.

[6] Ballantyne (1892).

[7] This is discussed later in the meeting (see page 35).

never treated a case of erythroblastosis fetalis; they had no training in serology or genetics. So how did this unlikely group manage to tame a terrible disease and bring this episode in medical history to such a satisfying conclusion? There are many dimensions to the Rh story and it would be wonderful today to have some light shed on at least some of them. So, Professor Weatherall, we are in your hands.

Weatherall: Thank you for setting the scene so nicely for us. At the beginning we ought to at least try to get some general background about the evolution of interest in blood group genetics and serology in the UK. I think there would be nobody better to help us than Professor Pat Mollison. Pat, can you lead us off?

Professor Pat Mollison: Yes. It has already been pointed out that one of the first labs in this country working on blood groups was the Galton Laboratory Serum Unit set up by R A Fisher with Rockefeller money in 1935.[8] In 1937, by a lucky chance, Rob Race, a young pathologist destined to become a great figure in blood grouping, was appointed to help G L Taylor. They worked for the first few years only on ABO and MN,[9] which were (apart from P) the only blood group systems known at the time, although from the early 1940s they started on Rh – and I will say a word about that in a moment. Meanwhile, in 1940, there were four London transfusion centres,[10] and the one I worked at, which was at Sutton, was extremely interested in blood groups. People working there did some very useful work on dangerous universal donors.[11] We had a very

---

[8] The MRC Blood Group Unit succeeded the Galton Laboratory Serum Unit, set up in 1935 under the direction of Professor (later Sir) Ronald Fisher and financed through the Medical Research Council by the Rockefeller Foundation. The Serum Unit was based at University College London and re-located to Cambridge during the Second World War. In 1946, the Unit was reconstituted at the Lister Institute of Preventive Medicine as the Blood Group Research Unit, under the directorship of Dr Robert Race (until 1973), Dr Ruth Sanger (until 1983), and followed by Dr Patricia Tippett. The MRC Blood Group Unit moved from the Lister Institute to premises at University College London, in 1975 and was disbanded in September 1995.

[9] Professor Patrick Mollison wrote: 'The MN and P blood group systems were discovered in 1927 by Landsteiner and Levine by injecting human red cells into rabbits and testing the resulting antisera against panels of human red cells.' Note on draft transcript, 4 August 2004.

[10] The London Blood Transfusion Service was established in 1921. For a history of blood transfusion services in the UK, see Dodsworth (1996); Gunson and Dodsworth (1996); Giangrande (2000).

[11] Professor Patrick Mollison wrote: 'Group O subjects are "universal donors" in the sense that their red cells can safely be transfused to almost everyone. However, the plasma of a small number of group O subjects ("dangerous universal donors") contains potent anti-A or -B, which, if transfused to group A, B or AB subjects, may cause a haemolytic reaction.' Note on draft transcript, 4 August 2004.

bright physician, John Loutit from Australia who, with others, carried out very interesting experimental work in human subjects. It would be quite impossible to do that now, of course; very little was done in the way of getting permission.

Early in 1942 the US work on Rh became known in the UK. At that time we had a Canadian physiologist, Omond Solandt, who, unlike me, read journals. He told me that he had seen an article by Levine and that I should take an interest in it.[12] Meanwhile we were sent some guinea pig anti-Rh from Landsteiner's lab. It was a terribly bad reagent and was extremely difficult to work with. The obvious solution was to find a woman who had had a baby with haemolytic disease. I went over to the Mayday Hospital in Croydon in March 1942, and found a woman whose serum agglutinated eight out of the ten samples tested with it. I gather that Rob Race did much the same in Cambridge, at about the same time. From then on, we were able to do Rh grouping. It was possible to diagnose haemolytic reactions due to Rh incompatibility and to diagnose Rh haemolytic disease, because one could find the antibody in the mother. A lot of other laboratories during the early stages of the war were interested in transfusion. For example, the first example of anti-c was found by McCall in Stoke on Trent, Cappell in Glasgow found anti-C, and Boorman and Dodd in Sutton found anti-E.[13] Race by this time had taken over from G L Taylor as Head of the Galton lab, and everybody sent their samples to him. Fisher was still in London at that time as Professor of Genetics at UCH but he became Professor in Cambridge in about 1943. He used to go down and see Race regularly and look at his results. There was a famous day in the pub called the Bun Shop when Race showed him his latest results. Fisher came up the next morning with his 'CDE' idea: the idea that Rh antigens are determined by three closely linked pairs of allelic genes.[14] In the USA the same Rh specificities were encountered, but it was postulated that they were determined by multiple alleles at a single locus. One great advantage of the 'CDE' concept was that everybody could talk about it so easily.

Until 1945 the only method of detecting blood group antibodies was by agglutination in saline, which detected IgM antibodies. As all immune blood

---

[12] Levine *et al.* (1941).

[13] McCall and Holdsworth (1945); Race *et al.* (1943, 1944).

[14] A description of Fisher's reasoning can be found in Fisher (1947); see also Race and Sanger (1982). Professor Patrick Mollison wrote: 'An alternative form of a gene is an allele; every cell has two sets of chromosomes and therefore two copies of any particular gene, one inherited from each parent.' Note on draft transcript, 4 August 2004.

group antibodies are, at least partly, IgG, they couldn't be picked up unless they happened to have an IgM component.[15] It wasn't until 1944 that Race demonstrated what he called an 'incomplete antibody':[16] incomplete Rh antibody would attach to cells, and stop them from being agglutinated by other anti-Rh antibodies. Almost immediately afterwards there was a flood of tests that would detect IgG antibodies. Most famously, Coombs, working with Race and Mourant in Cambridge, developed the antiglobulin test.[17] Diamond and Denton in Boston discovered the agglutination-enhancing properties of albumin as a medium, and Pickles in Oxford showed that enzyme-treated red blood cells were agglutinated by IgG antibodies.[18] These discoveries opened up the field tremendously. From about 1945 onwards, one could detect so many new antibodies and one blood group system after another was discovered.

The only other thing I wanted to comment on is that once blood group antibodies could be identified so easily, many strands of interest developed. There was the biochemical approach, particularly by Morgan and Watkins on the ABO and Lewis systems;[19] there were the genetic linkages between blood group systems, the first one perhaps was between MN and Ss, picked up by Race and Sanger.[20] Then there was the association between blood groups and disease. I think the first there was possibly Ian Aird, the surgeon, who identified the strong association between blood group O and peptic ulcer.[21] Then there was the difference of frequencies of blood groups in different races, for example the increased frequency of D-negatives in the Basques.[22] From the clinical point of view, there were incompatible reactions and the whole question of haemolytic disease in the newborn to be investigated.

---

[15] Professor Patrick Mollison wrote: 'Antibodies are immunoglobulins (Ig) and may be IgA, IgG or IgM; naturally occurring blood group antibodies are usually IgM and immune antibodies usually IgG. Only IgG antibodies are transferred across the placenta from mother to fetus.' Note on draft transcript, 4 August 2004.

[16] Race (1944).

[17] Coombs *et al.* (1945a, 1945b). Note that C Moreschi in 1908 discovered the principle of the method [Moreschi (1908)]. See also Mourant (1983); Tansey *et al.* (1997).

[18] Diamond and Denton (1945); Morton and Pickles (1947); Pickles (1989); See also Pickles (1949).

[19] Morgan and Watkins (2000).

[20] Race and Sanger (1975): 92–138.

[21] Aird *et al.* (1953, 1954).

[22] Nijenhuis (1956–7).

Weatherall: Thanks very much for starting us off so well. Dr Beryl Corner, would you like to fill in on some of that?

Dr Beryl Corner: The Army Blood Transfusion Service was set up in 1939, at the onset of the war, by sheer chance in the grounds of Southmead Hospital in Bristol.[23] Southmead Hospital then opened a very large maternity department with 140 beds altogether, and the Medical Officer of Health for Bristol (Professor R H Parry), a very progressive man, had arranged antenatal clinics all over the city, and means of antenatal blood testing for women in the city. Colonel Lionel Whitby was in charge of the blood transfusion service and from the beginning he offered his services to any clinicians in the area who wished to use them. So as soon as the rhesus factor had been discovered, as we have already heard, by Wiener and Levine,[24] Lionel Whitby began to include this test on the blood that he examined from donors. So he had the rhesus typing established. By 1943, all bloods coming from antenatal patients in the area had rhesus typing performed on them by Whitby and his group. Geoffrey Tovey was the lieutenant there who was responsible for all this. In 1943 our first case of Rh haemolytic disease was diagnosed and treated by Geoffrey Tovey and myself: a three-hour-old baby, born in a local maternity hospital, and a very, very sick baby, pale, with bruising and petechiae all over. Geoffrey Tovey established that this was in fact a case of Rh incompatibility. The baby was far too sick to contemplate cutting down on the veins, which would have been necessary in those days, with the primitive equipment available, and so I actually treated the baby directly into the bone marrow. I gave about 50 ml of Rh-negative blood into various places of bone marrow and saved the baby's life. That patient survived and was followed up by us, and when he was aged 18 he became a blood donor, rhesus positive.

The other thing I would like to say is that I spent a day at Aldershot in 1990, at the blood transfusion service there, and I went through the archives of all the correspondence and all the papers that had been collected by Lionel Whitby and Geoffrey Tovey and the correspondence with the War Office. I got some statistics about blood transfusions that had been done by the Army Blood Transfusion Service during the war. One of the interesting things was that they established an Rh-negative panel of donors, with 79 donors, up to 1945 and they also established donors for the other blood groups as well, but

---

[23] Whitby (1944).

[24] See note 4.

they had actually a Rh-negative panel of 79 donors at that stage. At that time, of course, we knew nothing about exchange transfusion, but we were regularly treating babies who were diagnosed as having haemolytic disease, and we were treating them just with straight blood transfusions. We reckoned that we cut the mortality by 50 per cent for haemolytic disease due to Rh incompatibility.[25]

Weatherall: Thank you very much indeed. Just a matter of technology: was intramedullary transfusion, that is transfusion straight into the bone marrow, a standard practice for neonates at that time?

Corner: No, it wasn't. The problem was that there were no suitable needles small enough to put into veins of babies, and any transfusion attempted in 1943 on a baby meant a cut-down needle, and inserting an adult-sized cannula, and that particular baby was in no state for that procedure.

Weatherall: What we have heard from Pat [Mollison] is a bird's-eye view of the development of knowledge about the genetics, the early diagnostic testing, the importance of the Coombs test and so on, and the kind of first stuttering approaches to treatment. Is there anybody else who would like to say anything about that particular period – that is, the further development of knowledge about the genetics of the system – and what you were thinking at that time, or the idea of preventing this disease, given that you knew about the basic pathophysiology very clearly at that time? Were there any thoughts about prevention for the future?

Mollison: I think the idea of artificial insemination from Rh-negative men was certainly discussed.[26] It was quite a lively topic at one time.

Weatherall: That was your idea was it?

Mollison: No, no.

Dr Derrick Tovey: I was going to carry on from Dr Beryl Corner because I went to Bristol to work with Geoffrey Tovey, and it is important to realize that

---

[25] Corner (1947). Professor Maureen Young wrote: 'The use of exchange transfusion for the treatment of infants with rhesus incompatibility in the early years after the Second World War provided physiologists with the opportunity to study the infant's cardiovascular reactivity.' Further details are provided in a brief paper provided by Professor Young and will be deposited with the records of this Witness Seminar in Archives and Manuscripts, Wellcome Library, London.

[26] See, for example, Bregulla (1978); www.baccweb.com/serv_art1.htm; www.radmid.demon.co.uk/rhesus.htm#choices (sites visited 24 September 2004).

we were doing exchange transfusions every day. There were, in fact, two or three mothers every day in England and Wales who lost a baby with Rh. An important factor in Great Britain was that most transfusion centres then tested all Rh-negative women for antibodies, and this allowed for many obstetric and paediatric centres, such as Bristol, Newcastle and Lewisham, to specialize in the management of these mothers and their babies.[27] I have one anecdote to add. While I was there, I had a phone call from a maternity unit in Gloucester asking if I wished to do a post mortem (pm) on a rhesus baby. I said I wasn't particularly interested in doing a pm, but when did it die? 'Oh', she said, 'It's not dead yet'. So I put the equipment in the back of the car, collected our nurse, and we drove up to Gloucester and did an exchange transfusion. I am only pointing this out because of the importance of having regional centres that were expert in this condition.

Corner: I should have added something to what I said just now. By 1945, every baby born under our service had its cord blood done, with all the grouping factors, and if the mother was Rh-negative, the Coombs test was done. By 1945, we were doing Coombs testing on all babies of Rh-negative mothers on blood from the umbilical cord.

Dr Timos Valaes: I want to go on with the story that Dr Corner, my mentor at the time, started. I joined the paediatric staff at Southmead Hospital in 1956. The excitement of treating erythroblastotic babies with exchange transfusion almost every day became the turning point in my professional life and led me to neonatology.[28] If I am allowed to continue a little on the subject, I consider the emergence of neonatology and, a little later, of fetal medicine as collateral benefits of the work done by people like Professors Mollison and Coombs, who provided the definitive tests for recognizing maternal isoimmunization and its consequence: haemolytic disease of the newborn (HDN). Things moved very fast. By the time the techniques for *in utero* interventions were fully developed, the advances in Rh disease prevention resulted in diminishing numbers of affected fetuses. By the 1970s a rhesus-

---

[27] Dr Derrick Tovey wrote: 'I mention Newcastle above because of the pioneer work of Professor "Willie" Walker and Dr Sheilagh Murray, then Director of the Newcastle Blood Transfusion Centre, who led the way in the centralized treatment of babies with Rh disease.' Note on draft transcript, 11 November 2003.

[28] Dr Sheila Duncan wrote: 'With the introduction of exchange transfusion in the late 1940s and early 1950s, it should be noted that not all problems were solved and that many cases died *in utero.*' From a letter to Dr Daphne Christie, 19 November 2003. See Diamond (1983).

negative young woman could be reassured that the probability of survival for her progeny was as good as that of a rhesus-positive woman.[29] This was an enormously brighter outlook for the lives of millions of prospective mothers and – I must add – fathers.

Weatherall: Thanks very much. What we have done, in a sense, apart from outlining the genetics, was to jump from the very first efforts of a kind of treatment to the time when exchange transfusion, intrauterine transfusions became more routine, and I wondered if it would be possible perhaps for Charles Rodeck to introduce this area and try to put it in a kind of temporal perspective for us at the moment, because we seem to have jumped straight from the very first primitive (if you might excuse the term) effort trying to get some blood into a baby to the time of well-developed technology of exchange transfusions.

Professor Charles Rodeck: Thank you. There are other people in this room who were in the field earlier than I was, and who, I hope, are going to contribute. But I think that as far as attempting to treat the problem while the patient is *in utero*, one of the first crucial steps was to refine diagnosis and prognosis, and to define who needed treatment and who did not. That meant making use of the knowledge that these babies became jaundiced and that the bilirubin levels were high in the amniotic fluid. Now, when this was being thought about, and the initial efforts were being done, an invasive procedure on the uterus was very, very rare indeed, and thought to be partly an invasion of a sacrosanct area, and partly also very risky. I think the name most associated with those early studies on bilirubin levels in the amniotic fluid is Douglas Bevis, who was working in Manchester in the early 1950s.[30] Then in the late 1950s and early 1960s there was William Liley in New Zealand who took it further and developed the charts for the assessment of prognosis.[31] He did

---

[29] See Clarke and Hussey (1994).

[30] Dr Sheila Duncan wrote: 'It wasn't actually bilirubin at first because it was not possible to measure this. It was blood pigments. The liquor amnii was known to be bright yellow in severe rhesus-immunized cases and Douglas Bevis's first paper on the subject [Bevis (1950)] measured iron and showed increasing amounts with severity, the liquor being obtained at the time of induction of labour. Later, he showed that non-haematin iron and urobilinogen taken at labour induction, at various gestations, correlated with severity [Bevis (1952)]. These studies led to liquor being obtained serially by amniocentesis to predict severity and help to time delivery [Bevis (1956)]. Chemical analysis was later refined and normal and abnormal values defined as intraperitoneal transfusion became established by Liley.' From a letter to Dr Daphne Christie, 19 November 2003.

[31] A Liley chart uses the spectrographic measurement of amniotic fluid bilirubin levels plotted against gestational age to estimate the severity of rhesus disease. See Liley (1961).

spectrophotometric measurements on the amniotic fluid to measure bilirubin and found that these were correlated with outcome. Many centres, of course, were working in this area by then and were starting to develop their own charts, and so the Liley charts, although they were probably the best known, were by no means the only ones. Again, some of the other people here might wish to comment on that.

With a method available to determine the severity of the condition, which was, I would say, reasonably accurate from late second trimester onwards into early third trimester, the next question was what to do. Early delivery so that the baby could have the benefit of exchange transfusions postnatally was the standard treatment and it had a great impact, but it still didn't help those that were too preterm to deliver and not yet viable. In those days, of course, neonatal units weren't prepared to accept infants born at 24, 25 or 26 weeks. The only option they had was to die *in utero.*

It was Liley again who then introduced the next major development. He did the first fetal intraperitoneal transfusion in Auckland, New Zealand, in 1963.[32] Very rapidly, many other centres around the world took this up. It was a highly courageous and risky intervention, because ultrasound guidance wasn't available then.[33] There was only one's sixth sense and a friendly radiologist who might want to get involved and take X-rays after injection of contrast media into the amniotic cavity. It had quite a high mortality rate, partly because it was reserved only for the sickest babies. Despite that, it spread around the world. I believe the first transfusion in this country was done by Mrs Jadwiga Karnicki at Lewisham. As soon as she heard of Liley's success, she whizzed off to New Zealand, and it was a case of 'see one, do one, teach one', I think. That was then the era of intrauterine treatment with intraperitoneal transfusion for almost 20 years.

Weatherall: Okay, so phase one, we are talking about intrauterine transfusion. Are there other people who have reminiscences or memories of what sounds like a fairly hairy period of development?

Corner: I think we have jumped a bit, if I may say so, because exchange transfusion was the big breakthrough, and this was first described by the Boston group in the USA in 1946. Our first three exchanges were done by

---

[32] Liley (1963).

[33] This was the subject of a previous Witness Seminar, 'Looking at the Unborn: Historical aspects of obstetric ultrasound'. See Tansey and Christie (2000).

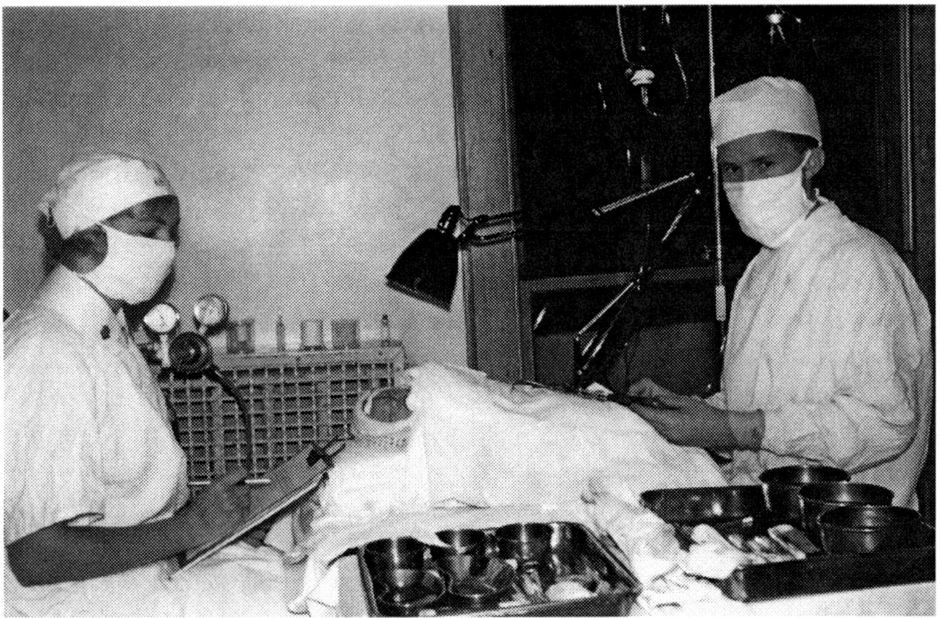

Figure 1: John Walker-Smith as an obstetric senior house officer in 1961, performs an exchange transfusion on a newborn with haemolytic disease due to rhesus incompatibility at the King George V Memorial Hospital, Sydney. Walker-Smith (2003).

Geoffrey Tovey and myself in 1948. Then exchange transfusion became routine treatment for babies diagnosed with haemolytic disease and other jaundiced babies as well during the 1950s (see Figure 1).[34] It was not until the 1960s that the intrauterine transfusion was well developed,[35] when it was realized that, although exchange transfusion was saving a great many babies who were born at birth with obvious early signs of haemolytic disease, hydropic babies could not as a rule be saved by that means. Therefore the endeavour was made to find means of getting to the hydropic babies before they became hydropic. In other words, this led to the desire for fetal transfusion and in the early 1960s this started.

Zallen: What was the success rate of the exchange transfusions? Do you have an estimate of how many babies survived and how many were lost?

---

[34] See, for example, Diamond *et al.* (1951); Diamond (1983).

[35] See, for example, Liley (1963).

Corner: Yes. When the exchange transfusion techniques really became established, which was during the 1950s, the survival rate was very high indeed. By 1955 we had exchanged well over 100, with 146 term infants, or near-term, and 16 premature babies as well. So it was a very high survival rate at that time when we got the technique really established. Our biggest problem then, in the 1950s, was the lack of laboratory facilities, especially micromethods that could give rapid results on small quantitites of blood for estimating bilirubin in the newborn infant, because the decision as to when to exchange depended on an estimation of the rate of rise of bilirubin to the point where it could cause kernicterus – kernicterus then became the subject that was being researched during the 1950s. I myself wrote a paper on kernicterus and prematurity, which was published in the *Lancet* in 1950,[36] in which we examined the deaths from hyperbilirubinaemia of premature babies. This was also the principal cause of death of the babies with haemolytic disease due to rhesus or other blood group incompatibility, for example ABO; that also came to light at this phase in the 1950s. When we discovered kernicterus we realized that this had got to be prevented by blood exchange, before the bilirubin in the blood rose too high, but our biggest problem was the lack of laboratory facilities for estimating serum bilirubin quickly. Bilirubin in severe cases had to be estimated two or three times in 24 hours, and we needed instant results, not results the next day, which was what most laboratories were capable of doing at that time. So in the 1950s this was an enormous stumbling block to the progress for treatment of this disease.[37]

Dr Archie Norman: I came into the rhesus field later than Beryl, and I have much less experience than she has. Mine was very much that of the plumber, with some advisory role as well. But, in order to come here today, I dug out my 1954 edition of *Recent Advances in Paediatrics*, and read Mollison's chapter there, which is, I think, excellent, and covers the whole field.[38] His conclusions there were all rather tentative. I then picked up the 1958 edition and read Lathe and Claireaux's chapter[39] in which almost all of what Mollison had suggested had been confirmed, and by then the use of estimations of bilirubin for controlling hyperbilirubinaemia and preventing kernicterus were almost, or were, routine. In

---

[36] Aidin *et al.* (1950).

[37] Corner (1958).

[38] Mollison and Cutbush (1954): 110–32.

[39] Lathe *et al.* (1958): 87–124, 125–44.

addition, exchange transfusion had become accepted. At that time I did most of the exchanges at Queen Charlotte's Hospital, London, and, I must say, an exchange transfusion even then was a matter of some anxiety. In about 1951 Lathe had said in his paper that it was a matter of great concern.[40] To get a rather firm plastic catheter into the umbilical vein of a small, perhaps anaemic and rather ill, baby was not always easy, and the estimations of the amount of blood you gave them also needed care. Towards the middle or latter end of the 1950s, soft vinyl catheters came into use and that made life very much easier, together with the two-way tap. So exchange transfusions became, I think, considerably safer and much easier to perform.[41] At the Royal Society of Medicine, I managed to find the Queen Charlotte's Hospital reports from 1950 to 1960 and found that there was a steady fall in mortality, a steady fall in kernicterus, but no change in neonatal deaths. Now that was probably because we were using early induction of labour more, so that there was a shift from the stillbirth rate to the neonatal.

I found that dealing with rhesus problems was emotional and stressful. Not only was there the problem of what one was going to do, but also of collaboration with the obstetricians.[42] When I first went there, we were not on the easiest of terms with the obstetricians, who saw little use for paediatricians. Fortunately, once we had begun to do the exchange transfusions, they felt they had got rid of something they weren't too keen on. Furthermore, we had a very friendly collaboration in the question of when and if to do an early induction.

I have little else to say, except that one can forget so easily, I think; I don't know how many of the practising doctors present have ever seen a case of kernicterus, but it's a dreadful condition. And for the woman who had already lost one baby, or who had a severely affected baby, to go through pregnancy and labour again is extremely stressful and one became very closely associated with them during that time. As a result, when one was able to produce a healthy baby, after exchange or otherwise, I found that the gratitude from parents was very much more marked than for almost any other condition I had dealt with. From my own point of view, maybe irrelevant but a thing that I have never forgotten, was driving home in the early morning after an emergency

---

[40] Lathe (1955).

[41] Walker and Neligan (1955). 250 cases between 1947 and 1954 are described using polyethylene catheters.

[42] This is discussed in one of the previous Witness Seminars, 'Origins of neonatal intensive care in the UK'. See Christie and Tansey (2001): 12, 26, 27.

exchange, and that feeling of elation that one really has done something for once. It was great.

Mr Elliot Philipp: Dr Karnicki has been mentioned. She published three separate papers on intrauterine transfusion,[43] but she did it under the stimulus of a man who has not been mentioned today and that is Alistair Gunn, obstetrician at Lewisham Hospital, who was her senior colleague. Now the difficulty with preterm delivery was inducing labour so that the risks of prematurity and the baby dying from prematurity would not be as great as those of dying from the rhesus disease, kernicterus and so on. Alistair Gunn became quite an expert at assessing weight just by palpation. He was quite remarkable at it, and it was he who persuaded Dr Karnicki to do intrauterine transfusions. They, I think, were the first non-teaching unit (at Lewisham) to do exchange transfusions,[44] and they taught me to do them. I did a very large number of them too, and I agree absolutely with Dr Norman, that it is a very hazardous and nerve-wracking procedure; and you drove home after doing them with a great sense of satisfaction.

Dr Jean Smellie: I don't have anything like Dr Corner's or Dr Norman's experience, but I was able to observe the change in attitude to exchange transfusion after its early introduction and also the effect of the many man-hours spent by paediatricians on exchange transfusions, often needing repeats.

The first 'exchange' I saw was on Christmas Day 1949 when I was an undergraduate on the 'list'. It was well remembered because after it I walked from UCH to Waterloo, to attend (rather late) a family lunch where a sceptical medical uncle said, 'Well, it won't do any good anyway, will it?'. This was very much the general attitude to erythroblastosis and exchange transfusion at that time.[45]

However, the figures for St Mary's Hospital, Manchester, for the three years from 1949 up to 1952 (when exchange transfusion was well-established) showed a dramatic reduction in kernicterus and fetal loss, among 90–100 mothers with rhesus incompatibility per annum. The UCH figures for much smaller numbers for the decade from 1949 to 1959 – involving 116 mothers, the majority with a previously affected fetus/infant – showed a similar effect. Two of the seven neonatal deaths that occurred were during exchange

---

[43] See, for example, Altmann *et al.* (1975a, 1975b).

[44] Berriman (1971).

[45] Diamond (1947, 1948).

transfusion; there were 12 stillbirths and none of the 97 survivors had kernicterus. Not surprisingly, when the gestation of these pregnancies at the time of delivery was related to outcome, the risk of hydrops increased with length of gestation and the risk of neonatal respiratory problems increased with early induction of labour. So these were major reasons for seeking some means of preventing the condition.

Professor James Scott: A small point related to kernicterus, which we referred to, and Grant Lathe's work at Queen Charlotte's. I came across Lathe at Charlotte's in 1951, 1952, and I met up with him again in Leeds in 1961. At a funeral more recently – which is where most of my encounters are! – I re-introduced myself to him and he said, 'Good God, I thought you were dead!' As far as I know *he* is still alive, at least he was two months ago, and a resident in Leeds. I think it would perhaps be a pity if he weren't contacted to make a contribution to whatever comes out of this, because he was right at the centre of the work on kernicterus.[46]

Mr Humphry Ward: I am simply going to add to what Charles [Rodeck] has said, although I think we have perhaps jumped a little bit ahead, because I think one of the key obstetric landmarks was the use of amniocentesis. I think it was Walker who suggested that it was pointless planning amniocentesis much before 34 weeks, because there was nothing that paediatricians could do to save these babies. It is fascinating to look back at Liley's original data and read his closing paragraph, because it sums the whole thing up. He says, 'The aim of the exercise, that is of intrauterine transfusion, is simply to arrest deterioration if possible and gain a few extra weeks of gestation, so that the skilled paediatric care of severe haemolytic disease is not nullified by gross prematurity'.[47] That was the key thing, of course, about Liley's work. I should say that I had the privilege to work with him in the middle 1960s and he was the most remarkable man. He was a person who knew everything; there was no topic that he didn't have an opinion on. He was a very humble man actually, and he never wanted to boast about what he considered was such a simple principle of physiology that he was putting into practice. At the time he was a senior research fellow, but he then became a Professor of Physiology, neonatal physiology, I think, actually. He was a wonderful man.

---

[46] See, for example, Lathe (1955); Lathe *et al.* (1958). For a biographical note see page 78.

[47] Liley (1963): 1109.

Professor Charles Whitfield: You mentioned, Mr Chairman, that the early uterine transfusions were hairy procedures. The same things applied to exchange transfusion. The first exchange transfusion was in 1946 by Wallerstein in New York.[48] He used the sagittal sinus to put in the blood and he drained it from a peripheral vein. Even before that, 20 odd years before, in Toronto, a man called Hart had done a similar case: a lady had a succession of stillbirths, and I have seen the notes of gross oedema and although it wasn't then recognized as a case of rhesus, it clearly was. My first contact with exchange transfusion, since we are reminiscing, was in 1949 as a student in Belfast, when I was hauled in to assist with an exchange transfusion and my job was to keep a count of the blood taken out (this was measured), and also to wipe the clots with a wipe or cotton wool (I can't remember), so that the outflowing blood could be measured in a galley pot; the transfused blood was given through a vein exposed by a small incision at an ankle (in the then usual way). That baby lived. Then in 1954 I got to Malta and within a few days was doing an exchange transfusion with glass cannulas and bits of metal linked together with rubber tubing, and with just a two-way syringe. The Henderson syringe with three-way flow (in, out, and for the blood) made a huge difference in this experience we have mentioned. Later on, the better plastic catheters also made such a huge difference, and the procedure ceased to be a nightmare.

Weatherall: What you have been describing is an extraordinary learning curve, from the mid-1940s through the following ten years, which relied not only on technical skills, but also on interaction with the laboratory, on the development of better methods for measuring bilirubin (also, presumably, the identification of critical bilirubin levels at which babies were at risk of kernicterus), and also on the ability of the laboratory to produce appropriate blood for exchange. Where were these fundamental, important bits of clinical research done? Were a number of them done in this country?

Mollison: We did produce evidence that kernicterus didn't occur with serum bilirubin levels of 18 mg per decilitre or less,[49] and this figure proved to be a useful guide.

Weatherall: What about these other technical developments, particularly the actual equipment and technique, the ability to deliver these transfusions? You

---

[48] Wallerstein (1946).

[49] Mollison and Cutbush (1951).

are saying that there were better needles, very simple things like that. How did these developments come about?

Corner: There was enormous pressure from the few paediatricians who existed in the 1950s and who had found their way even into maternity departments. We literally moaned and groaned to our biochemists that something must be done. But it was very difficult to get something done because in the 1950s, in the post-war phase of development of laboratories throughout the country, biochemists were very concerned with mass production of results of tests for electrolytes for instance, and to have to produce an urgent bilirubin result on a baby, where 5 ml of blood was what we were asked for very often, was something that was a bit tiresome, to tell the truth. I have rather sad memories of senior registrars standing at the telephone most of the day in the 1950s trying to get a bilirubin result back from a teaching hospital laboratory because they just had not been able to put it through with the techniques that they had at that time for doing it. I always say that the biggest advances in paediatrics came from plastics and electronics: plastic tubing for everything, including drip feeds and IV treatment, and then electronics in the equipment for getting quick results.

Coombs: Could I just point out that Wiener's technique of using an albumin solution to demonstrate haemagglutination did give positive results mostly – but Wiener was wrong in calling this agglutination 'conglutination'? That term had been given to a phenomenon first described in 1906 by Bordet and Gay, and whose mechanism was clarified by Bordet and Streng in 1909.[50] It involved a heat stable component of bovine serum named conglutinin, which caused the clumping of sensitized red blood cells, usually sheep or ox cells, in the presence of a non-haemolytic complement. In diagnostic laboratory tests, a conglutinating complement absorption test has similar uses to a haemolytic complement fixation test.

Dr Sheila Duncan: I think it's quite important to put the 1950s and 1960s into some sort of context from the obstetricians' point of view. Exchange transfusion was certainly an option after 34 weeks. Yet, even when it became more secure and successful, there was still a big problem for the obstetrician because so many of the more severely affected babies didn't make it to 34 weeks, as we have said. The perinatal meetings at that time were absolutely dominated by rhesus immunization. There were also preterm babies and babies

---

[50] Bordet and Gay (1906); Bordet and Streng (1909).

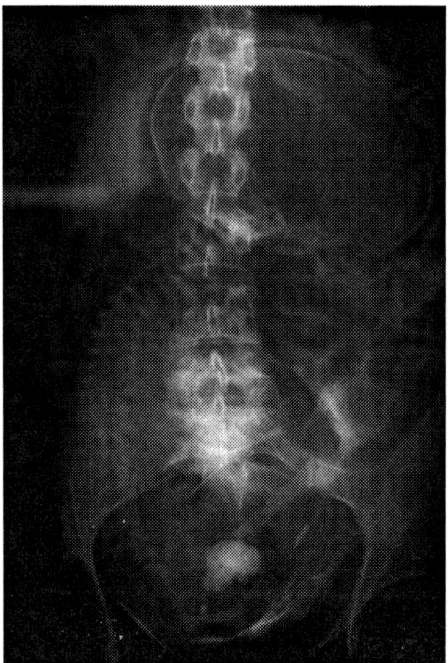

Figure 2: Radiograph taken on day after amniocentesis for bilirubin assessment and followed by contrast (1975). Swallowed contrast outlines the fetal gut, as well as remnants still in amniotic fluid. The delineation helped the insertion of the Touhy needle into the fetal abdomen. The fetus was in the breech position.

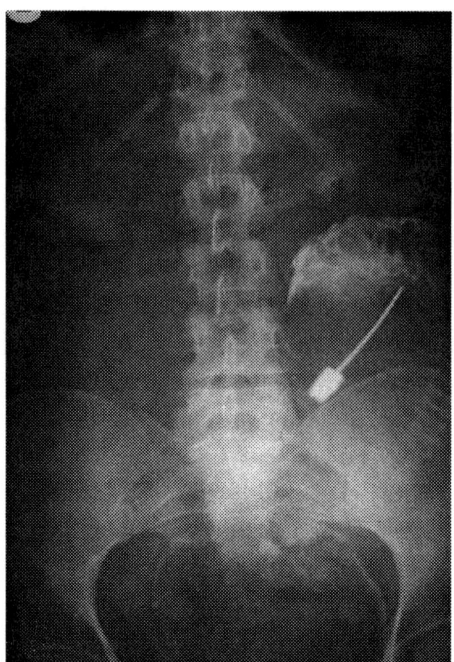

Figure 3: Touhy needle inserted into the fetal abdomen (1975). Some obstetricians fed a catheter into the fetal abdomen and gave the blood slowly. Others (as here) relied on the needle and gave the blood over about 20 minutes.

with congenital abnormalities, but it was the rhesus cases we thought that we could perhaps do something about. The severe intrauterine cases of rhesus disease were extremely important and sometimes dramatic, because if a woman had a severely affected baby who died *in utero* well before 34 weeks, she often retained that baby *in utero* for some weeks. Usually she had had previously affected babies and this was the end of the line. Indeed her safety was at risk because there wasn't much idea of inducing labour at 30 weeks with a dead baby at that time. When she did labour, she was subject to DIC (disseminated intravascular coagulation), or afibrinogenaemia as we called it then, and her life was in some danger. So, the prospect of intrauterine transfusion was really

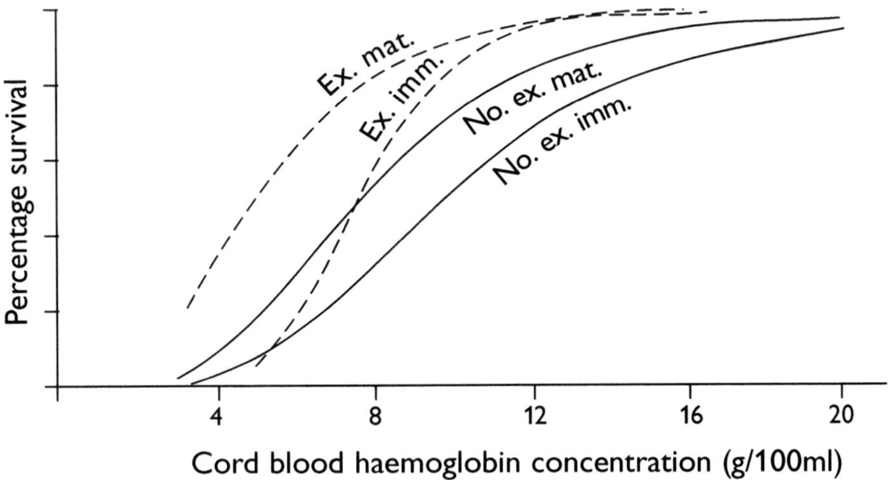

Figure 4: Curves relating the haemoglobin concentration of cord blood to the chance of survival, with different forms of treatment. Ex, exchange transfusion (sometimes less than 50 ml blood/lb body weight); No Ex, simple transfusion or no transfusion; Mat, mature, that is born at term or within ten days of term; Imm, immature, that is, born 35–18 days before term. Redrawn from Armitage and Mollison (1953). See note 51.

very important. The success rate was low at the beginning and, when it began to be used more widely in the mid-1960s, the failure rate was still really quite high. But in the severe cases, diagnosed by amniocentesis and using Liley curves, there was more to gain than to lose. The technique gradually developed, and this I think should be commented on. Amniocentesis was done, and some contrast was injected, which the fetus swallowed, so that within 24 or 48 hours when you had the amniocentesis result and the blood was available and you were ready to do it, the baby had outlined its gut.

The techniques by today's standards were extremely crude. X-ray screening helped to locate the needle in the peritoneal cavity (see Figures 2 and 3). A little contrast medium could be injected to identify this positively. I have seen many pictures of IVPs, cystograms, and the contrast in various cavities, but nevertheless even with the 30 or so per cent success rate, which I think is what it was in the early days, gradually increasing, they were very rewarding situations. But there was still a high fetal loss rate. It also sometimes stimulated labour and although that was unfortunate, the alternative was sometimes worse and I think this area of activity should be recorded.

Valaes: I want to remind the audience that the only multicentre randomized trial on the treatment of Rh hemolytic disease of the newborn was done in England.[51] It convincingly demonstrated the superiority of immediate exchange transfusion over simple transfusion so that the issue was settled once and for all. Early exchange transfusion was considered important not only for theoretical reasons but for a practical issue as well. With the stiff nylon tubing used to catheterize the umbilical vein, the success rate for later attempts was low (this has already been mentioned by Dr Norman).[52] The criteria for deciding that treatment was needed were based on the level of cord blood haemoglobin. In terms of the multicentre clinical trial, this study was again a first for establishing the need for careful standardization of critical laboratory measurements – in this case haemoglobin. When, appropriately, the emphasis shifted to bilirubin measurement and, if necessary, repeat exchange transfusions, the lack of satisfactory standardization of bilirubin measurement plagued the management of neonatal jaundice. This is a problem not totally resolved even now. I hope that Professor Mollison will forgive me for taking the words out of his mouth.

Tovey: Just to put into perspective all these new techniques; in 1950 the deaths per 1000 births in Britain was 1.6; by 1970 when you had exchange transfusion, amniocentesis, premature deliveries, intravenous therapy, it had dropped only to 1.2 deaths per 1000 births. Five years later, it went down to 0.4. Of course, what happened in 1970, we all know; we will hear later. But it is interesting that the total deaths per 1000 births didn't drop terribly much in that period of time 1950–70 (see Figure 5).[53]

---

[51] Mollison and Walker (1952); Armitage and Mollison (1953), see also Figure 4. Professor Patrick Mollison wrote: 'The figure summarizes some of the results of the controlled trials of treatment referred to by Dr Valaes. In infants not treated by exchange transfusion, the chance of survival was inversely related to the cord blood haemoglobin concentration. At all degrees of anaemia in mature infants, survival rates were greatly increased by exchange transfusion.' Note on draft transcript, 4 August 2004.

[52] See page 15.

[53] Tovey (1984): 100. See also Clarke and Mollison (1989). Dr Sheila Duncan wrote: 'A considerable proportion of the fetal losses due to rhesus immunization were stillbirths or deaths before 28 weeks which would not be included in the figures. Even after 1970, it was many years before already immunized women had finished child-bearing.' Note on draft transcript, 27 September 2004. Professor Derrick Tovey wrote: 'Although the measure prior to 1970 when anti-D prevention was introduced did result in a slow decline in infant deaths due to Rh it was only after the introduction of Rh prophylaxis that a dramatic fall in infant deaths occurred.' Letter to Dr Daphne Christie 1 October 2004.

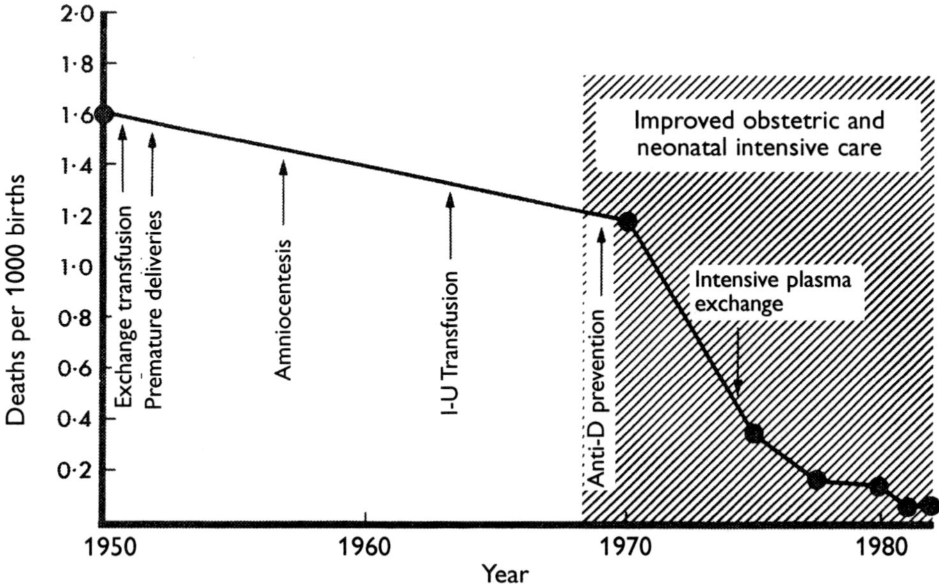

Figure 5: Perinatal deaths due to anti-D haemolytic disease of the newborn per 1000 births. Adapted from Tovey (1984): 100.

Weatherall: I think that's an excellent point to start moving on. Pat Mollison set the scene in a sense, in starting to ask the question that Doris Zallen addressed at the beginning and that was 'why Liverpool?'. As Pat pointed out, in the early development of human genetics, particularly medical genetics, the blood groups were really the only markers, and it was therefore almost inevitable that anybody who became interested in genetics in the 1950s would at least be thinking about blood groups. Maybe that's not the reason, but John Woodrow is going to try to give us some background about how these things might have started to develop in Liverpool.

Professor John Woodrow: I speak with some trepidation, because I feel that the ghost of Cyril Clarke is going suddenly to appear among us, and tell us how it all really happened. It is reported that J B S Haldane used to say in the 1930s and 1940s that in the whole world there were only about half a dozen people who knew much about human genetics, and all but one of those were Englishmen.[54] The work of these pioneers was carried out either in London or

[54] See Kevles (1995): 205. The people include Haldane himself, Fisher, Hogben, Penrose, with the non-British one being the Swede, Gunner Dahlberg.

not many miles from London and it was some time before involvement in research into human and clinical genetics spread to other parts of the country. In the case of Liverpool it was not until the mid-1950s[55] and this came about because of a seemingly minor event, that is the appearance in 1952 in the *Amateur Entomologists' Bulletin* of an advertisement from Philip Sheppard of the Department of Zoology in Oxford, seeking pupae of the swallowtail butterfly *Papilio machaon.* Cyril Clarke responded to this and it is worth reflecting on the fact that this exchange was to have a profound effect, not only on their lives but also on those of several people who are present today. Cyril had recently discovered how to hand mate swallowtail butterflies and had carried out some experimental crosses between two related species. The two soon met and began their collaborative work on the genetics of Batesian mimicry. Cyril's enthusiasm and energy and Philip's expertise in genetics together with his scientific rigour, proved to be a powerful combination. As far as I am aware, Cyril had not previously had any particular interest in human genetics, but the possibility of working together in this area was discussed and Philip suggested 'blood groups' as a basis for a programme of clinical research.[56]

Why blood groups? On his return from the war Philip had gone up to Oxford in 1946 to read honours zoology. There he came under the influence of E B Ford and subsequently obtained his DPhil on the population genetics of butterflies and snails. Ford was much concerned with the evolution and maintenance of balanced polymorphism. He had worked with Ronald Fisher who over the years made major contributions to several areas of human genetics. Fisher, as has been already mentioned, set up a blood-grouping laboratory at the Galton Laboratory in 1935.[57] There were three areas in which the blood group polymorphisms played an important role in the study of human genetics in the early decades of the century.

Firstly these polymorphisms were the only basis for testing the new ideas on population genetics as exemplified by the works of Hardy and Weinberg and this led, for example, to the clarification of the genetics of the ABO locus by

---

[55] See Zallen (1999): 197–216.

[56] A very brief account of the prevention of Rh haemolytic disease is given in a recording of Professor Philip Sheppard, 18 March 1968, available in the Genetics Society Archive (1968; SID I, 1–180), John Innes Centre Archives, Norwich.

[57] See note 8.

Felix Bernstein in 1924.[58] Secondly was the question of genetic linkage. There was a wish to emulate the achievements of the *Drosophila* geneticists and establish genetic markers on as many chromosomes as possible. It was hoped that the slowly increasing list of blood group polymorphisms might provide a basis for this and thus enable clinical geneticists to furnish a more exact prognosis for individuals in families affected by mental deficiency, Huntington's chorea etc. There was the possibility of detecting the heterozygous carriers in conditions such as Friedreich ataxia and phenylketonuria. The first to provide a satisfactory method for determining linkage was Bernstein in 1931[59] and he was followed in this by Hogben, Haldane, Fisher and Penrose. The early attempts to demonstrate linkage proved disappointing and it was not until several decades later that real progress became possible.

The third application of blood groups was with regard to the possibility of population associations between blood groups and clinical disorders. It is worthy of note that this question was being investigated as early as 1917 at the Mayo Clinic in Minnesota and some negative results were published in 1921.[60]

We now return to E B Ford in Oxford, who in 1945 suggested that a search for population associations between the ABO and secretor polymorphisms and disease might well be productive.[61] Philip Sheppard would have been well aware of this and so it is not at all surprising that when he began working with Cyril Clarke the opportunity was taken to initiate such studies. Much work along these lines was carried out in Liverpool in relation to peptic ulcer, rheumatic fever etc. but the results did not lead to any major advance in our understanding of disease causation.[62]

The work on Batesian mimicry in swallowtail butterflies at first suggested that the variation of wing pattern which allowed for the mimetic forms to evolve, was based on a series of alleles at a single locus.[63] However, further experiments

---

[58] Bernstein (1924).

[59] Crow (1993).

[60] See, for example, Buchanan and Higley (1921).

[61] Ford (1945).

[62] See, for example, Aird *et al.* (1953, 1954).

[63] This was discussed in an interview with Clarke arranged by the Royal College of Physicians and the School of Biological and Molecular Sciences, Oxford Brookes University, UK. 1986. See Sir Cyril Clarke in interview with Sir Gordon Wolstenholme, 15 May 1986 (Medical Sciences Video Archive 610.695/CLA). Oxford: Oxford Brookes University.

strongly favoured the existence of a group of closely linked loci with a particular group of alleles, which constituted what Darlington and Mather had referred to as a 'super-gene'.[64] Several years previously the complex serology of the Rh antibodies had been gradually revealed, and provided a challenge to those attempting to understand the genetic structure of the Rh system. Pat Mollison has told us how Fisher put forward the concept of three closely linked loci and this proved very useful in practice and was widely accepted.[65] There was one person who bitterly and persistently disagreed with this interpretation and that was Alex Wiener. He insisted on a proprietary right to the Rh system of blood groups, in particular that the Rh antigenic specificities resulted from the presence of a series of alleles at a single Rh locus and that his nomenclature should be the only one used. His somewhat vituperative letters and diatribes directed at Rob Race were well known in Liverpool, and I think Cyril admired the great forbearance displayed by Race. Cyril and Philip thought that there was a parallel between the Fisher–Race model of Rh genetics and that of Batesian mimicry and this led in turn to an interest in Rh haemolytic disease of the newborn.

A remarkable feature of Batesian mimicry is that it is only expressed in females, and this implies that the genetic determinants of maleness are suppressing the expression of the genes involved in mimicry. In other words there is gene interaction. Philip Levine had reported in 1943 that when he studied a group of Rh immunized mothers, there was a lower than expected frequency of instances where the father was ABO incompatible with the mother, for example father group A and mother group O.[66] This finding received support from the experimental work of Curt Stern who injected ABO-compatible and incompatible RhD-positive blood into RhD-negative subjects and confirmed the protective effect of ABO incompatibility.[67] Later Nevanlinna showed that the pregnancy that induced primary Rh immunization was usually the one that preceded the first affected child and that in the great majority of instances the child in this pregnancy had been ABO compatible with the mother.[68] One can calculate that of all immunized mothers, approximately only 1 in 35 had been initiated by an ABO incompatible pregnancy.

---

[64] Clarke *et al.* (1968).

[65] See page 6.

[66] Levine (1943).

[67] Davidsohn *et al.* (1956); Stern *et al.* (1961).

[68] Nevanlinna and Vainio (1956).

It was considered that the interaction between the Rh and ABO systems was 'similar to' the interaction between the genes determining sex and those determining mimicry in the swallowtail butterflies.[69] I will stop there because Ronnie Finn is going to tell us what happened next.

Weatherall: That's really set the background very nicely.

Zallen: If R A Fisher hadn't hypothesized a cluster of loci or a 'super-gene', do you think that the Rh locus would have attracted any interest in Liverpool? I just wondered because Wiener, of course, was very insistent that his model of one locus with many alleles, and his notation, be accepted. If that had been the case, there might not have been the idea that the Rh locus was something like the butterfly locus responsible for mimicry.

Woodrow: When Cyril Clarke and Philip Sheppard initiated the studies concerning the possible association of blood groups and disease, there was no particular interest in the Rh groups. Cyril, in his paper in *Scientific American*, after describing the genetics of mimicry in butterflies, states that 'we could not help noticing certain striking parallels between the inheritance of their wing patterns and inheritance of blood types in man' and then goes on to refer to the Fisher/Race model of the Rh system.[70] If the latter had not been previously described, it seems unlikely that Cyril's attention would have been drawn to the Rh groups and thus to Rh haemolytic disease of the newborn and to the protective affect of ABO incompatibility.

There is I think one lesson that the controversy between Fisher/Race and Wiener teaches, and that is that such controversies are usually not solved by further polemics but by advances in knowledge, which in turn are often the result of applying new technologies. Thus one had to wait for advances in molecular biology before it became possible to make progress in understanding

---

[69] Professor John Woodrow wrote: 'The process of Rh immunization depends in the first place on the *relationship* between the Rh alleles of mother and fetus, that is the mother must have no RhD alleles and the fetus must be heterozygous RhD. A secondary determinant of Rh immunization is the *relationship* between mother and fetus at the ABO locus such that where the mother is, say, group O and the fetus is group A, the risk of immunization is much decreased. In neither mother nor fetus is there any interaction between the Rh and ABO loci. This is in contrast to the situation in Batesian mimicry where in the *individual* butterfly there is interaction between the male determining locus and the cluster of loci determining mimicry. That being said, the view may be taken that in the light of history, the important thing is that the attention of Cyril Clarke was drawn to the protective effect of ABO compatibility.' Letter to Dr Daphne Christie, 27 November 2003.

[70] Clarke (1968).

the genetic structure of the Rh system and this is work that is still continuing.[71] There are people here today who can update us on that.

Weatherall: But it hadn't been. I saw Ronnie Finn shaking, or by his standards, fiercely shaking his head a moment ago, so maybe we should hand over to him. Ronnie, did you chaps really start work on rhesus in this logical way, knowing that this gene cluster might be like the butterfly cluster?

Professor Ronald Finn: Not really. I first became involved in this when I was SHO (senior house officer) to Cyril Clarke.[72] I wanted an MD thesis, and he said to me, 'You can work on the interaction between ABO and rhesus blood groups'. I knew nothing about either, and I was immediately dispatched down to the Lister, to Dr Mourant's laboratory, to learn how to hold a pipette and how to do blood grouping. To watch a physician holding a pipette must have been a funny sight at the time. ABO incompatibility, in mating, is defined as one in which the father is unable to give blood to the mother. An example of such a mating would be an A father and an O mother. If the mother is also Rh negative, and the fetus Rh positive, then any ABO incompatible Rh-positive fetal cell that enters the maternal circulation will be destroyed, or inactivated, and Rh sensitization prevented. Thus, as Professor Woodrow has already said, Levine had discovered that ABO incompatibility between mother and fetus protects against rhesus disease,[73] and it was Race and Sanger who suggested that the incompatible cells were destroyed and, with them, the rhesus antigen was also inactivated in some way.[74]

My project was simply to provide further evidence in support of ABO incompatibility as a protective mechanism against Rh disease,[75] and I had to carry out family studies on families with and without rhesus disease. The important point was that working on a daily basis with ABO incompatibility as a natural protective mechanism against Rh disease probably inevitably led us to speculate as to whether other protective mechanisms could be devised. We knew about ABO incompatibility. We knew the main protective mechanism

---

[71] See Clarke (1968).

[72] Background of the Liverpool work is given in Clarke and Finn (1977). See also Zallen (1999).

[73] Levene (1943).

[74] See Race and Sanger (1950).

[75] Finn *et al.* (1961); Longo (1977). See also Professor Ronald Finn's statement on Rhesus factor at the symposium on the role of inheritance in common diseases held at the Liverpool Medical Institution on 18 February 1960, in Anon. (1960).

was the placental barrier, but we were on the lookout whether there was another way of doing it. The obvious way was to find some way of mimicking ABO incompatibility. The difference between maternal and fetal red blood cells in this situation is that the fetal red blood cells are Rh positive and the maternal red blood cells are Rh negative. Therefore, we suggested that an Rh antibody, anti-D, would be expected to either selectively destroy, or inactivate in some way, Rh-positive fetal cells without damaging the Rh-negative maternal cells and so protect the mother against Rh disease. Thus, the hypothesis was stimulated by ABO incompatibility. It was, in a very simple sense, a copy or mimic of this natural protective mechanism.

The hypothesis was then tested in Rh-negative male volunteers by injecting Rh-positive blood to produce Rh sensitization. We tried to block it with anti-D. Initially we used saline agglutinating antibody or 19S, as a direct copy of ABO incompatibility. But this did not protect. In fact, it made matters worse and we changed to 7S-antibody which was highly successful. We initially used high titre pooled anti-D, but later changed to anti-D gammaglobulin, mainly to reduce the risk of serum hepatitis. The red blood cells were labelled with radioactive chromium to study clearance, which we used as an index of coating with antibody.[76]

The use of passive anti-D was, however, only part of what was called the Liverpool hypothesis. The generally accepted view at the time, put forward by Levine, was that fetal cells leaked through the placenta intermittently throughout pregnancy, and he thought that sensitization could occur at any time, probably from three months onwards. This conventional view would mean that anti-D would have to be given on several occasions, including relatively early in pregnancy. We were concerned that this would cross the placenta and might cause the very disease that we were trying to prevent. We now know, of course, that anti-D can be given safely during pregnancy, but we did not know that at the time, and we were certainly very worried about giving it to a very small fetus, where we might produce problems. Therefore the second part of the hypothesis – they both stood together or fell together – was that sensitization was usually a focal event in time, and usually occurred at delivery. This suggestion fitted in with the work of Nevanlinna, who pointed out that rhesus disease was unusual in the first pregnancy and suggested that sensitization took place in the first Rh-positive pregnancy and that overt

[76] See Finn *et al.* (1961): 7.

disease occurred in the next Rh-positive pregnancy. We had simply extended the concept of a sensitizing pregnancy by suggesting that most significant transplacental haemorrhages were associated with trauma to the placenta during delivery, which was eminently logical.[77] If this was correct – and this is the main point – large doses of anti-D could be given after delivery without any danger at all to the fetus. In order to test this hypothesis we used the Kleihauer technique,[78] which had become available about a year or so previously, to study the incidence and timing of transplacental haemorrhage, and it was demonstrated that most significant bleeds were associated with delivery, although much smaller bleeds did occur, mainly in the latter months of pregnancy. This finding supported the suggestion that sensitization usually occurred at delivery, but the final proof would require clinical trials in Rh-negative mothers given anti-D only at delivery, and that comes later.

Can I finish with one or two general comments? Number one, serendipity, as so often in research, played a large part in this work.[79] We did not start off with the intention of preventing Rh disease. Once we got involved with a protective mechanism, we stumbled on it. Number two, the initial and critical first step was to copy the natural protection afforded by ABO incompatibility. That's what the whole thing was. Again I want to emphasize that the Liverpool hypothesis had two parts: the use of passive anti-D to inactivate the fetal cells and, secondly, the concept of delivery sensitization.

Finally, I must say that this was very much a team effort; it involved a lot of people over a considerable time. As Professor Woodrow, Dr Towers, and myself are the only ones here today, I think I should briefly mention the others. Dr Dermot Lehane was Director of the Liverpool Blood Transfusion Service. All the male volunteer studies were carried out in the Blood Transfusion Service. Without him, it could never have happened. Dr William Kulke provided the chromium-labelled cells. We were very fortunate in Bill Donohoe, who was a brilliant blood-group technician, Dr Richard McConnell was Cyril Clarke's chief-of-staff who monitored the whole thing. He was my MD supervisor and he was the one who suggested the use of 7S, rather than 19S antibody when that had failed. Philip Sheppard, whom Professor Woodrow has already mentioned, was Professor of Genetics, and he advised us on experimental

---

[77] Wiener (1948).

[78] Kleihauer *et al.* (1957).

[79] See Tovey (1992). This is a recurrent theme that has come up in other Witness Seminars.

design and statistics. Finally, last but by no means least, the charismatic leader of our team, Sir Cyril Clarke, who had the uncanny knack of making things happen. No matter what Wiener had said, or did not say, Cyril Clarke would have gone in this direction, I have no doubt. If Cyril Clarke had not suggested that we work on ABO incompatibility as a protective mechanism, the whole thing would never have happened. His remarkable journey from butterflies to rhesus certainly deserves a place in medical history.

Weatherall: Thanks very much, Ronnie, for that remarkably succinct description of the long period of research. With so many interesting lessons, or perhaps non-lessons, developed in medical research in that short story, I think that it is worth spending a few moments thinking about some of them. May I start off with a question, Ronnie? Why did Cyril suggest that thesis project to you? It was pretty well known what the answer would be, wasn't it? For anybody outside the British scene, you should know that in those days you had to take a postgraduate research degree for an MD, to be respectable. Why do you think he suggested that problem?

Finn: It certainly had nothing to do with prevention, I think it was just a project that would lead to an MD thesis. And the other point was that we could strengthen the evidence by looking at the sensitizing fetus. In an ABO-incompatible mating, the father could be homozygous or heterozygous, and if he was heterozygous then the next fetus could be ABO-compatible, and, therefore, you could get a lot more evidence to support that hypothesis if you looked specifically at the ABO-incompatibility status of the sensitizing fetus. That was the specific point.

Weatherall: Just one more quick question before I throw this open. The kind of serendipity of timing is always so important and the ability to identify fetal cells in the maternal circulation is very important here. My memory is that the Kleihauer paper came out in about 1955 or 1956, and then the paper of Alvin Zipursky in Toronto.[80] Was it his group who first actually showed the value of it for detecting fetal cells in the maternal circulation?

Finn: Yes. It was about 1956 or 1957, and I started in 1958, so we were very, very fortunate. As you were saying before, whatever the theory says, you have got to have the right technology, and it came along for us just at the right time.

---

[80] Kleihauer *et al.* (1957); Zipursky *et al.* (1959); Zipursky and Israels (1967). Professor Ronald Finn enclosed an illustration of fetal cells erythrocytes in the maternal circulation in a letter to Dr Daphne Christie, 25 November 2003. This will be deposited with the records of this Witness Seminar in Archives and Manuscripts, Wellcome Library, London.

Woodrow: Ronnie Finn did part of the experimental work in Baltimore where I followed him after a year. It is interesting to look back at the way the experimental studies in RhD-negative male volunteers were conducted respectively in Liverpool and Baltimore. Dermot Lehane was the key figure in this regard in Liverpool, where his blood donors had the greatest trust in him. It was in an atmosphere of simple altruism that the work was carried out in the Blood Transfusion Centre or at places like Vauxhall's factories or the petrochemical factories in Ellesmere Port and so on.

Such volunteers were not available in the USA where it was common practice to use prisoners for medical research. In Baltimore the 'volunteers' for the experiments were inmates of the Maryland State Penitentiary, where the liaison was organized by Julie Krevans, head of the Johns Hopkins Hospital Blood Bank. The prisoners used to receive, as I remember, a pack of cigarettes and US$3 for each injection or sample of blood. This use of prison inmates was forbidden under subsequent legislation.

Weatherall: Would you like to enlarge on just what those were? What were you doing in a penitentiary or what was Ronnie doing in a penitentiary? What were you doing to these 'volunteers'?

Woodrow: The studies in Baltimore were integrated with those in Liverpool. Groups of six RhD-negative men were injected with small volumes of RhD-positive blood and half in each group were then given varying amounts of plasma containing anti-D with varying characteristics, the procedure being repeated up to four times. In some experiments survival of the ^{51}Cr-labelled red blood cells was measured. All the volunteers were subsequently tested for the development of an anti-D response. In summary, it was found that plasma containing high titres of 'incomplete' anti-D rapidly cleared the injected red blood cells to the spleen and was very effective in suppressing the active anti-D response.

Some interesting light was thrown on the immune response to RhD-positive red blood cells in that in some control subjects, decreased survival of the cells was found for weeks and sometimes for months before any anti-D could be found in their serum.[81] Thus a primary response could occur without antibody being detectable by serological methods. In others, survival of repeated injections of red blood cells was normal and they appeared never to develop anti-D.

---

[81] Mollison (1970).

May I add a little to what Ronnie has said about transplacental haemorrhage (TPH)? Study of maternal blood samples taken immediately before and immediately after delivery suggested that where evidence of TPH was found after delivery, in about two-thirds of such cases this had probably occurred quite recently. Ronnie and I looked for evidence of TPH in 398 blood samples taken at various times during pregnancy. In 6.3 per cent of samples there was evidence of an increase in maternal HbF (fetal haemoglobin) which made it impossible to detect the presence of fetal cells. Evidence of TPH was found in 3.5 per cent of samples taken during the third trimester but not earlier in pregnancy.

Returning to the penitentiary, there was a story I heard when I went to Baltimore after Ronnie had returned to Liverpool, that he used regularly to have his hair cut by one of the volunteers, who turned out to be in prison for homicide.

Weatherall: Ronnie, you had better enlarge on that statement.

Finn: I was only a research fellow on an NIH (US National Institutes of Health) grant at the time and we didn't have much money. My hair had got longer and longer and I could not afford to go to have a haircut, so the senior nurse in the hospital wing where we worked in the penitentiary suggested that she would have it cut for me. I said OK and it was very necessary at the time, because my hair was relatively long (it's not long now of course) and the Americans were going through the crew-cut stage. So they locked me up in a little cage, which was about ten or 12 feet square, with this chap who cut my hair. The hair at that time went down the back of my neck and he got his cut-throat razor out, down the back of my neck. He suddenly stopped and he said, 'Do you know, they have never let me have an open blade?' He looked like a gangster and if he walked in here now we would all line up against the wall. But being in Hopkins, they dealt with him. They got the psychologist to see him, and they got the plastic surgeons to fix his nose and pull his ears back.

Weatherall: Thanks, Ronnie. Can we move back to rhesus now?

Dr Barry Benster: I wonder if I could make a very personal comment on the use of anti-D in the prevention of rhesus disease? I'm a retired obstetrician from West Yorkshire but, more important than that, my blood group is O rhesus-positive and my wife Sonia is O rhesus-negative. In 1968, I was what was called an exchange senior registrar in Malta and our daughter was born there at the naval hospital, and I believe that my wife had the first injection of anti-D immunoglobulin, which was flown out by courtesy of the RAF in 1968. I can't claim that we went on to have another 15 or 20 children, as many of the Maltese women did at that time, but our next child was born without any immunization.

Tovey: Can I ask a question of you Liverpool people? As you know, the Americans – Freda, Gorman and Pollack – worked on the concept that in the presence of passive antibody the giving of the antigen prevented active immunization in a very specific way.[82] The Liverpool workers based their researches on the concept that the fetal Rh-positive cells could be removed from the maternal circulation; this would prevent sensitization. I would like a comment on the fact that since we had been giving anti-D when I was working in Leeds, we found there was no decrease in any other antibody produced by the mothers. You would expect that if, in fact, the mechanism of protection were by simply removing fetal cells, you would get a reduction in other antibodies, but we never found that.[83]

Weatherall: Would anyone like to comment on that?

Woodrow: I am not sure whether Derrick Tovey is referring to RhD-negative mothers who have been treated with anti-D. Of course non-Rh antibodies would still be appearing in some RhD-positive mothers and as the incidence of anti-Rh antibodies fell, the former would constitute an increased proportion of all antibodies found. I am not aware of any published data that documents the development of non-Rh antibodies in treated mothers and I would be very surprised if their development were other than a very rare event. You will remember the Liverpool 'anti-Kell' experiment in which 62 D-K- volunteers received two successive stimuli with D+K+ red blood cells, with half also receiving anti-K immunoglobulin. Eleven of the 31 controls developed anti-D but only one of the 31 given anti-K did so.[84] This suggested that immunosuppression with IgG antibody was antigen non-specific. There is still some uncertainty as to the actual mechanisms involved in antibody-mediated immunosuppression and a very interesting seminar could be held around this.

---

[82] Pollack *et al.* (1968a); Freda *et al.* (1977).

[83] Dr Derrick Tovey wrote: 'After a discussion with Professor Woodrow I have re-examined the data that I presented in my paper [Tovey (1986)], where I reported the number of Rh-negative mothers receiving anti-D prophylaxis had shown no decrease in the incidence of other than anti-D antibodies (see table V of that paper) and as a result questioned the "Liverpool" theory that anti-D protects by simply removing fetal cells from the maternal circulation, because if this were so one would expect a reduction in the numbers of antibodies to all blood group antigens in the fetal red cells. A deeper analysis of our finding however does not merit such a confident prediction as the two major antibodies reported, namely anti-E and anti-Kell were probably either "naturally occurring" or due to blood transfusion and therefore independent of a sensitizing process to fetal red cell antigens.' Letter to Dr Daphne Christie, 1 December 2003.

[84] Woodrow *et al.* (1975). For a review on anti-Kell in pregnancy see Leggat *et al.* (1991).

Weatherall: Pat [Mollison], would you like to say anything on that? Not really, I see. So you are still arguing that after all this time the mechanism is not clearly understood. I think it's rather a critical point for this meeting.

Dr Patricia Tippett: When I was working in Boston in the 1950s, they were trying an immunological protection by desensitizing the women who had lost affected babies. Dr Allen was injecting his own R_0 blood (Rh-positive phenotype) which he knew was OK and he hadn't had jaundice or anything. This, of course, didn't succeed in protecting any of these women, but there was one case where a woman made an additional unrelated (anti-Kidd) antibody.

Dr Belinda Kumpel: Just a quick word about the anti-D or the mechanism of immune suppression that may be happening. It's not really known for certain, although earlier on in the 1960s and 1970s there were some nice experiments done on rabbits[85] by several of the people here, and since then on mice as well.[86] However, none of the experimental animals are suitable models for Rh-D. This is because Rh-D negative people lack the whole molecule as they do not have the Rh-D gene, whereas rabbits have a true polymorphism of a blood group and make allo-antibodies. Mice have no blood groups. So xenogeneic cells are used, usually sheep red blood cells, and both the antibodies that are formed are different. In mice it's usually IgM. The timing of antibody appearance suggests the mechanisms are different in the three situations as well.[87] So it is very difficult to actually solve it with humans,[88] because you can't ask for samples of spleen from volunteers, which is what would be required.

Zallen: I would like to ask about the comments that Cyril Clarke made that this was a group of amateurs.[89] Was the team really such a group of amateurs? Did they start as amateurs and become more polished researchers?

Weatherall: Perhaps we had better hear from both of them. We might then get some kind of balance.

Finn: Cyril Clarke always described himself as an amateur scientist, and I think that fitted in with us at that time. The main point was that we weren't involved

---

[85] Pollack *et al.* (1968b); Elson *et al.* (1971); Smith and Mollison (1974).

[86] Heyman and Wigzell (1984); Karlsson *et al.* (1999).

[87] Kumpel and Elson (2001).

[88] Combined study (1966); Pollack *et al.* (1968a); Kumpel *et al.* (1995).

[89] Zallen (1999).

in Rh or blood group work; we weren't from the laboratory; we weren't blood transfusion people; we weren't paediatricians; we weren't obstetricians and we weren't immunologists. So we were completely divorced from the ordinary way of doing things.

Weatherall: If that's not a good definition of an amateur, what is?

Finn: But in a way often that is better because, if you are coming from completely out of the field, you can think laterally, whereas people within the field find it much more difficult.

Weatherall: Pat, what did people who were really in the field think in the early 1960s about this approach?

Mollison: Well, I don't think they were confident it was going to work.

Weatherall: Why?

Mollison: Just general scepticism, I suppose, not very rational. I think everybody accepted the idea that ABO incompatibility prevented or diminished the chance of Rh immunization. I don't think there was general confidence that immunosuppression using anti-Rh was going to work, and I don't know why that was.

Weatherall: Johnnie [Woodrow], did you want to comment on the amateuristic atmosphere in your laboratory at that time?

Woodrow: That is a rather complex question. The technology was pretty unsophisticated but we had an excellent serologist in Bill Donohoe, and those involved in the fetal cell counts went to great pains to make the method as accurate as they could. The experimental design of the experiments was far from amateurish. I am always struck when I go back to the published papers (and this also applies to the 'blood groups and disease' studies) by how carefully and generally well-written they were and they certainly do not read as the work of amateurs. The people involved differed from each other in various respects as was to be expected and it was the great achievement of Cyril Clarke and a tribute to his powers of leadership that they worked so well together over a period of several years. It is also important to put on record here the contribution of Féo Clarke who was involved with Cyril's work at every level and who was, I am sure, an indispensable collaborator in all aspects of his research activities.[90]

---

[90] See Weatherall (2002).

Finn: I would certainly agree with that. She was a remarkable lady. In her eighties she went to the Open University and learnt to speak Russian so that she could read Russian novels in the original language. Just to follow on from Professor Mollison, I think one of the reasons there was such great scepticism was we were altering completely the natural history, or the view of the natural history, of rhesus disease, and the thing was even if the anti-D worked, when would you give it? This concept of delivery sensitization took a lot of accepting. I think that was one of the problems.

Scott: It was the creation of the Cyril/Féo combination that was vital to the whole story.

Weatherall: I will tell you more about that during the interval.[91]

Dr Frank Boulton: I came on to the scene very late. I came to Liverpool in the mid-1970s, and was a registrar at the London in the early 1970s. It was from conversation with John Jenkins, and from his reminiscences (by that time it was all established) that I think that people were very afraid for the baby. There was a lot of concern that giving something to the mother might continue to make the baby even worse. So I think that's just one little point of reminiscence.

The other question, which I think Belinda [Kumpel] was hinting at a little bit though, is why did the 7S work and not the 19S? Indeed the IgM even seemed, Ronnie, to make it worse from what you say. Have there been any thoughts about that?

Finn: I don't think we know. Professor Mollison may wish to comment?

Mollison: I think that IgM antibodies which don't bind complement, like anti-D, have never been shown to destroy red blood cells *in vivo*, and therefore it's difficult to believe that they are concerned here. With Nevin's help, we purified IgM anti-D and tried in volunteers to see whether it would suppress immunization. Although at the time we concluded that IgM had destroyed red blood cells, later on it seemed to me much more likely that the IgM preparation was contaminated with a small amount of IgG, and that this was what had produced the effect. We couldn't have detected the amount of IgG antibody that was there, but we worked out that there could have been enough. So returning to the Liverpool experiments, I don't think that the IgM preparation they used, the agglutinating anti-Rh, was responsible for the

---

[91] Further discussion of the importance of Féo in Cyril Clarke's work is found in Weatherall (2002).

increased number of responders. I think it is conceivable that it was the same case as with us, that there were traces of IgG anti-D there, which augmented immunization. There is, in fact, some evidence that very small amounts of IgG anti-D when given with red blood cells do actually augment the response, although I think you have to say that the case is not proven. There is no completely convincing explanation of why in Liverpool they found that giving agglutinating anti-Rh apparently increased the number of responders. I think this is a mystery.

Professor Peter Harper: As one who came in from the outside to work with Cyril Clarke and colleagues in Liverpool in the later part of the 1960s, I would like to come back to this question about a group of amateurs. I think that the group as a whole, and Cyril in particular, were far from being a group of amateurs. They were outstandingly talented, and I think the reason why, or perhaps one of the reasons why they were able to take a step that hadn't been taken by others more immediately involved, was just that. They were able to stand back from the immediate and specific aspects of the field, whether this be serology, or paediatrics, or obstetrics, and look at it as a kind of research problem from first principles. Cyril, in particular, was very much a person of first principles. Because of his basic experience in genetics, partly through his links with Philip Sheppard, he was able, I think, to move from one situation to another in a way that perhaps people more immediately involved in the applications were not.

People are often a bit disparaging about the butterfly work, but in fact it is strikingly modern. Workers in genetics use model organisms all the time, and now in human genetics one shifts, as indeed Cyril did then, between one species and another without much trouble. We know the genomes are all very similar. I think Cyril may have chosen butterflies as a rather unorthodox model organism, and I am quite sure one of the reasons he chose them was because they were more enjoyable than something like *Drosophila* to work with. But they were very valuable nonetheless. I think he was able to approach this problem from the point of view of theory, as Ronnie Finn has said, and look at it very broadly and I don't think there was any 'amateurism' meant in a disparaging way. There was extraordinary ability of the research design and original thought, and Cyril imparted that to all the people who were working with him.

Dr Peter Hunter: Two points. One about lateral thinking and another about the wives of clinical scientists. In the genesis of serious innovations in medicine in the twentieth century, and particularly treatments, lateral thinking has been extraordinarily important. Although we now accept that it is easy to treat schizophrenia, psychiatrists played no part whatever in the origin of the treatment of schizophrenia, which was actually created by the people who first made drugs like largactil which were then used by a military anaesthetist in the armed forces of France as part of a system for preparing patients for operation. The doctor involved, Henri Laborit, suggested to psychiatrists in Paris that drugs like largactil should be tried as a type of sedative for a variety of psychiatric disorders.[92] When the first patients received them, the results were so startling that the nurses couldn't believe their eyes.

The second point is about the influence of wives of great clinicians. There is a longstanding tradition that biographies are called, for example, 'Marlborough, His Life and Times,' I think in some cases serious consideration should be given to the title, 'Dr X, His Life, His Wife and Times'.

Dr John Silver: It is with some deference that I speak like the spectre at the feast of the amateur approach at Liverpool. All has been portrayed as sweetness and light, but it was an extraordinary experience coming to work in Liverpool. I was appointed in 1965 to work in Liverpool as Consultant-in-Charge of the Spinal Injury Service for Merseyside, and some days before I was due to move to Southport I got an approach from John Goldsmith (renal physician), who suggested that I wouldn't have enough work running the spinal unit, and I should take on the chronic dialysis programme for the whole of Liverpool. I was a bit surprised. I had just put down my mortgage in Southport and I thought I would have more than enough to do to run the spinal injury service for Merseyside single-handed. Anyway, after some weeks I went across to see John Goldsmith and was delighted and surprised to see the renal physician who had been appointed: Ronnie Finn. It was an extraordinary kind of atmosphere, especially the way we plan today, to think that you could be appointed to one post and just *al fresco* take over something like the chronic dialysis programme for a whole region. Of course I didn't, and I think Ronnie Finn did, but I would like to know, with some deference, was your experience of renal disease the same as mine?

Weatherall: I am not sure we should embarrass Ronnie in public by answering that question [he had no comment]. Can I ask an alternate question, Ronnie, because it is getting close to tea, and I had to review all Cyril Clarke's work recently? I came across that extraordinary article in the *Scientific American*, an autobiographical

---

[92] See Tansey and Christie (1998): 133–205, in particular page 140. See also Tansey (1998).

account,[93] where he clearly states that the first concept in your group to give patients anti-D arose when his wife Féo woke from a deep dream in bed and shouted at the top of her voice 'give them anti-D'. Ronnie, you probably were the closest to that, do you think that there is any possibility that that was true?[93a]

Finn: David, I thought this might come up and I had never thought about it before. But three or four days ago I thought I had better put my mind to it, and I think it could well be true. I don't think Cyril would ever tell a lie. My hypothesis is that at the meeting of the Medical Institution in Liverpool in February 1960, when I first mentioned that we might consider preventing rhesus disease with anti-D, this was a throwaway remark at the end of the paper. It was a symposium on medical genetics in which there were five papers within a two-hour period, so it was all pretty rushed, and the rhesus paper was in the middle and it was just one throwaway remark at the end of it. My hypothesis is that it didn't register with Cyril at all; he didn't hear it. But then the next thing that would have happened is that Cyril decided to write this up, which eventually became terribly important because it gave us priority over the New York group. That's why it became important, but at the time it wasn't of course. And Cyril and Féo used to write things up together, but I suspect that very often Cyril said, 'I am busy today, Féo, you write it up'. Then Féo would have come across this sentence about preventing Rh haemolytic disease, and, being Féo, she would have thought about it and worked out what it meant, and then she would have told Cyril. It might well have been in the middle of the night, but as you know Cyril went to bed very early, so it could have been in the middle of the evening. The other point, of course, is that the report in the *Lancet* simply said that Rh disease might be prevented by the use of a suitable antibody. I looked at my typescript notes the other day, and that's what it said. Some people say that I used the word anti-D or rhesus antibody at

---

[93] Clarke (1968).

[93a] Professor Doris Zallen wrote: 'The issue of priority was raised in Zimmerman (1973): 291–2. In a strongly worded letter of response to Zimmerman (dated 11 September 1973), Cyril Clarke maintained that it was indeed Féo who first made the suggestion to him. In that letter, a copy of which exists inside the Zimmerman book held in the Royal College of Physicians library in London, Clarke also offers the view that the idea could have arisen simultaneously within the group. As Clarke wrote, "I say I gave Ronald [Finn] the idea, and he says he thought of it himself. Both may be true – as Philip Sheppard suggested in his letter to you – after all, the Americans had the idea independently". Philip Sheppard's recollection, mentioned in the Introduction to this transcript, about first hearing the idea from Clarke can be found in an oral-history audiotape, *c.* 1968, in the John Innes Centre Archives.' E-mail to Dr Daphne Christie, 3 October 2004. A copy of the letter from Sir Cyril Clarke to Mr David Zimmerman (11 September 1973), will be deposited with the records of this Witness Seminar in Archives and Manuscripts, Wellcome Library, London.

the time. I don't remember whether I did or I didn't and we just don't know. It is possible that Féo actually worked out what the antibody was. So I believe that the first time Cyril did hear the idea was from Féo. That's my hypothesis.

Weatherall: I think I see the new Director of the Wellcome Trust sitting here,[94] and I hope coming in at the end of this conversation he has now got a clear idea of how to plan the future of really important science. I think we had better break for tea.

We left off the story when the preliminary clinical trials, or the experimental study in human 'volunteers', provided what is called these days a 'proof of principle'. What we need to know from the Liverpool group, and I hope they will tell us a little bit along the way, is what was happening in New York. Johnnie Woodrow's going to introduce this and we have got several people here who are absolutely key in those trials, so it will be extremely valuable. John, would you like to kick off?

Woodrow: The clinical trials, following the events that Ronnie Finn told you about, started in May 1964.[95] RhD-negative primiparae who gave birth to RhD-positive ABO-compatible babies were entered into the trial. As there was still uncertainty about certain aspects of the natural history of Rh immunization by pregnancy, the opportunity was taken to study the control mothers carefully in order to learn as much as possible about this. It was confirmed, for example, that when a primary immune response occurs as the result of a stimulus of RhD-positive fetal cells late in pregnancy or during labour, this may manifest in some women by the appearance of anti-D in the subsequent months but in others antibody is not found until the later months of the next RhD-positive pregnancy, in most cases due to a second stimulus. It was found that the larger transplacental haemorrhages seemed more likely to induce an immediate antibody response, while the smaller stimuli were less likely to do so but more likely to induce priming without detectable antibodies. It was therefore decided that the success of immunosuppression by anti-D would be measured in the first instance by testing for anti-D six months after delivery, and that the mothers would be followed up and tested again at the end of the second RhD-positive pregnancy.

[94] Dr Mark Walport was a Governor of the Wellcome Trust for two years and was appointed Director on 1 June 2003. Sir David Weatherall retired as a Governor of the Wellcome Trust in 2000.

[95] See Mollison and Walker (1952). Professor John Woodrow wrote: 'The work books recording the day-to-day entries in the clinical trial together with those documenting the experimental studies in the male volunteers in Liverpool and with other relevant documents including correspondence, are deposited in the Special Collections and Archives, Sydney Jones Library, University of Liverpool, referenced 530.' Note to Dr Daphne Christie, 27 November 2003.

The first trial involved mothers thought to be at highest risk, that is those whose fetal cell count after delivery indicated approximately 0.2 ml of fetal blood in the maternal circulation. Approximately 1000 mg anti-D immunoglobulin was administered to alternate mothers after delivery. This trial was conducted in collaboration with centres in Sheffield, Leeds and Bradford, and Baltimore. Thirty-eight of 176 control mothers and only one out of 173 treated had detectable antibody at six months. This represented a 97 per cent reduction in immunization at this time. On testing at the end of the second RhD-positive pregnancy, 20 out of 65 control mothers and two of 88 treated had anti-D, a reduction of 93 per cent.

A second trial was later commenced in Liverpool which included the women who had not been included in the first, that is, those whose fetal cell count suggested less than approximately 0.2 ml of fetal blood in the maternal circulation. A single blood sample taken immediately after delivery does not in all cases tell one how much fetal blood has entered the maternal circulation. For example, when there has been a small transplacental haemorrhage in the weeks prior to delivery which has induced priming, followed by clearance of the fetal cells, there may be none present at delivery. This is one of the explanations for the occasional failure of anti-D to prevent immunization in mothers whose blood sample after delivery had shown no fetal cells. The treated group were given 200 mg anti-D.

Tests six months after delivery showed 13 out of 362 of the controls to have anti-D compared with none of the 353 treated mothers. At the end of the second RhD-positive pregnancy, 13 of the 127 controls had anti-D as against three of the 128 treated mothers. This represented a 78 per cent degree of protection. The confidence limits here are wide, and when more treated mothers were followed up, this figure rose to 90 per cent. In some instances the appearance of antibody in the pregnancy subsequent to the treated one may be due to primary immunization and thus only preventable by antenatal anti-D.

Weatherall: John, thank you very much. Ronnie or Shona, do you want to add anything, or Nevin, who was very much involved at that stage?

Finn: I personally took no part in the clinical trials, but I watched the results, obviously with great interest, and one of the things that surprised me was the very high success rate. If we were relying purely on delivery sensitization, which was the original hypothesis, we should have had a success rate of probably 70 or 80 per cent. So I don't think that delivery sensitization is the whole story, and I think it's likely that there is some form of depression of the immune response during pregnancy, and there's a lot of clinical evidence of this. Things like SLE (systemic lupus erythematosus) will get much worse after delivery and so on, and we did do some studies looking at lymphocytes in pregnancy and mixed lymphocyte cultures between mother and fetus and they were in fact diminished, down, in pregnancy. So the remarkable results of delivery treatment suggest that this thing is a little bit more complicated than just the cells coming over at that time.

Mollison: I think one should mention that by a lucky chance Nevin [Hughes-Jones] produced his method of quantitating anti-D in 1967.[96] Up to that time, all these early experiments were done on titre, which is not very reproducible, and it is very difficult to compare one sample with another. So it was very fortunate that this came out at that time and it was possible, as you may remember, to have control trials of dosage in this country two years later; the effect of different doses was compared, and that would have been impossible without a quantitative method. I was very happy that it happened at that time.

Dr Nevin Hughes-Jones: The agglutination method was incredibly inaccurate. In some surveys that we did, you would get about 100-fold difference, with different people doing titres. So that the only contribution made by that measurement, in terms of micrograms, was that by radioactively-labelling the anti-D molecule, it did make the assay more accurate.

Weatherall: Dr Bangham is with us, who was involved with this.

Dr Derek Bangham: First let me explain that I am a medical innocent of specialized haematology. My career has been concerned with biological standardization – the characterization and measurement of biological substances important in clinical and research medicine. This was the responsibility of the Division of Biological Standards at the NIMR (National Institute for Medical Research), and since 1972, by the NIBSC (National Institute for Biological Standards and Control).

Yes, we ran a study to assess the accuracy of that method (which was believed to measure milligrams of anti-D immunoglobulin) in assays of coded samples. When Nevin Hughes-Jones learned of the international approach he then readily collaborated with us.

The long-proven procedure is to prepare a large batch of selected material, ampouled in stable form, against which other preparations can be assayed in appropriate comparison biological methods. A pool of sera from naturally

---

[96] Hughes-Jones (1967).

immunized multipara was provided by the Blood Products Laboratory at Elstree by Bill Maycock. This was freeze-dried in some 2000–3000 ampoules at NIMR. An international collaborative study was run in which coded (that is, unknown) ampoules of this and several other preparations were assayed by 23 expert haematologists in 11 countries.[97] All their raw data results were analysed statistically at NIBSC. The report of the study was accepted by the WHO Expert Committee on Biological Standardization and the ampouled material was established in 1976 as the First International Standard for Anti-D Immunoglobulin, to define the International Units of activity. This has stood for 30 years and is only now being replaced.[98]

Various attempts had indeed been made to convert haematologists from stating their estimates of blood-typing sera in terms of 'titres' of their local serum to using international units by assays against a standard properly calibrated in international units. When commercial preparations (for example, anti-D) became licensed for clinical administration, it was essential to have attested the internationally accepted methods with which to control their potency and quality.

I am explaining all this to set the record straight and show how research on assay methods is evaluated internationally. So this is another example of biological standardization in which this country has led intellectually, scientifically, and in hard practice. Britain now looks after almost all international reference biologicals.

Weatherall: I just wonder, while we are on the subject of international collaboration, we have not said much about the Freda and Gorman team in New York who were racing you, if it was a race. I don't know if John or Ronnie, or any of you, would like to say a brief word about the American enterprise, and how interactive it was with the Liverpool group.

Finn: I first found out about it when I went to see Philip Levine, when I was working at Hopkins, and he said you must go up and give a seminar at Columbia on medical genetics, and I got there and gave the seminar. At the end of it, three young men [John Gorman, Bill Pollock and Vince Freda],[99] my

---

[97] Bangham *et al.* (1978); Bangham (2000): 130–1.

[98] Thorpe *et al.* (2003).

[99] Professor Patrick Mollison provided a photograph of Sir Cyril Clarke, John Gorman, Bill Pollock and others, taken at a rhesus conference, McMaster University, 28–30 September, 1977, which will be deposited with the records of this Witness Seminar in Archives and Manuscripts, Wellcome Library, London.

age at that time, came along and asked a lot of questions, and said, 'We are doing similar work'. That came as a complete surprise to me. But it became obvious that they were also working on it independently, but using a different theoretical concept. And, as we said before, it hasn't finally been worked out which one is correct.

The other thing that they did at that time was that Bill Pollock from Ortho[100] gave me a specimen of the gammaglobulin, anti-D gammaglobulin, which I used. Relations between us at a personal level were very good. Of course, John and I both worked at the Hopkins for a time, so Julie Krevans in the blood bank there played a part in this as well. Relations were good. I don't think we, at our level, ever really thought about it as a major race. I don't know what John thinks.

Woodrow: I fully agree with Ronnie. When I was in Baltimore I paid several visits to John Gorman in New York and there was always a pleasant and free exchange of ideas and experience. Everyone wanted the work to go well. I remember an excellent conference on Rh prophylaxis organized by Bill Pollack at Princeton. You will recall that John Gorman had come from Australia to work in the Columbia–Presbyterian pathology department and spent much time in the blood bank. He was browsing through a general textbook of pathology and came across a reference to Theobold Smith, who in 1909 was working on the induction of immunity with diphtheria toxoid.[101] He had found that if too much antitoxin were given with the toxoid, active immunity failed to develop. This drew John's attention to the possibility of immunosuppression by antibody. Even prior to this, two pupils of Paul Ehrlich had reported in 1900 that if ox red blood cells were injected into rabbits an antibody response resulted but if specific antiserum were given with the red blood cells, the antibody response did not occur or was very weak.[102]

Weatherall: I remember talking to John Gorman. They got held up at the beginning because they had trouble persuading the NIH that this was worth supporting. Then I thought, from my memory of the Liverpool days, that this must have been the most shoestring research ever done. You just paid for a few Kleihauers.

Finn: I am not aware that any grant at all was given for it. Registrars worked for nothing; the technicians, Bill Donohue was working in the department;

[100] The Ortho Research Foundation. See Freda *et al.* (1964).

[101] Smith (1909).

[102] von Dungern (1900).

and all the work done at the Blood Transfusion Service was voluntary. I think it was done on a shoestring.

Zallen: When did the Nuffield Foundation grant come?[103]

Finn: That came much later, when the clinical trials were starting.

Weatherall: So this whole programme and all the basic work was done without one grant. I think that probably is worth recording.

Rodeck: I would say that in all likelihood this so-called bunch of amateurs, if they had applied to the Wellcome Trust for funding, would have been rejected.

Weatherall: (I think the new Director has left, hasn't he?) Any other comments or questions or queries about that critical period of clinical trial? It is a wonderful story and the results, compared with most clinical trials, were devastatingly good, weren't they?[104] Quite extraordinary. In the short time that we have got left, we have two other items before asking Pat Mollison to put the Rh locus into its present perspective. It would be helpful, I think, since we didn't have the chance earlier, to have a very brief update on what's happened on the structural side and our knowledge of the locus, and also, presumably as the number of folk with anti-D naturally declined, what's happened since in terms of monoclonal antibodies and current questions of availability of anti-D and so on. Did your success actually create problems? Is David Anstee here? Yes. You have several of your colleagues here and there have been major advances in our understanding of the rhesus system since we left off in about 1960.

Professor David Anstee: The critical experiments that opened up the route to identifying the structure of the protein were made by Stephen Moore, who worked in the Edinburgh centre of the Scottish Blood Transfusion Service,[105] and at the same time independently by Carl Gahmberg in Helsinki in 1982, when they showed that they could immune-precipitate the Rh proteins.[106] Having identified the proteins, then it was a question of applying the existing

---

[103] Professor Doris Zallen wrote: 'In October 1963, the Nuffield Foundation awarded Cyril Clarke and his group a grant of £350 000 to establish the Nuffield Unit of Medical Genetics at the University of Liverpool Medical School. This grant made possible the construction of a building and the support of many different lines of research on medical genetics. See Zallen (2002).' Note on draft transcript, 19 August 2004.

[104] Clarke *et al.* (1966).

[105] See Gridwood (1990).

[106] Gahmberg (1982).

technology to obtain enough of those proteins for some amino acid sequence determination and then to isolate cDNA.[106a] At about the same time, monoclonal anti-D was becoming available from the culture of B lymphocytes transformed with Epstein-Barr virus. Nevin was involved in that work in Cambridge, and Belinda Kumpel, who is also here, in Bristol. They provided enough antibody to purify sufficient protein for sequence characterization. So I think it was about 1990 when that process produced full-length cDNA for the first of the Rh proteins. That was obtained in Jean-Pierre Cartron's group in Paris and in our own group by Neil Avent, who is sitting in front of me.[107] So we had amino acid sequence for one of the Rh proteins derived from the cDNA sequence. By that time, we knew that there were at least two Rh proteins from immune precipitation studies. Subsequently it emerged that there were two genes: one that encodes D and the other that encodes C and E. I think that's rather a satisfying result, following on from the discussion earlier about the disagreement across the Atlantic between the Wiener hypothesis that there was one gene and the Fisher–Race hypothesis that there were three genes, because the right answer turned out to be there are two genes and so they were both wrong.

That characterization in 1990 established the nature of the proteins that give rise to the antigen and since then a great deal of work has been done to characterize the nature of the polymorphisms that give rise to the variety of antigenic structures upon those proteins. I think that was the critical phase: the identification of the molecules themselves by Stephen Moore and Carl Gahmberg originally, and then the cloning of the genes around 1990. D was cloned around 1993, the first cDNA sequence encoded the product of the CE gene. These findings formed the basis for all the work that has gone since.

Professor Neil Avent: I was involved in the cDNA cloning. Gene structures have been purported to be correct as the two Rh genes, which are in reverse orientation to each other, are on chromosome number one. If you look at some of the recent Sanger contigs, they don't actually totally agree with that idea. So the idea that the human genome sequence is complete, I think, is premature, especially in Rh genetics. So there's a little bit of work to be done looking at the correct orientation of the Rh genes and I think that this may vary between different Rh genotypes. If you look at one of the Sanger contigs, it encodes the big CE protein, which we all

---

[106a] Professor David Anstee wrote: 'A small segment of the amino acid sequence allows the synthesis of oligonucleotides that can be used to probe a cDNA library for a full length cDNA encoding the amino acid sequence of the whole protein.' Note on draft transcript, 13 September 2004.

[107] Cherif-Zahar *et al.* (1990); Avent *et al.* (1990).

know is extremely rare and very unlikely. On a closer analysis it is half of a RhD gene and half of a RhCE gene (Rh-D, Rh-CE). So this contig is not correct. I still think that more work is needed to look at the genomic arrangement of Rh genes in different Rh genotypes and work out what precisely is going on, because I don't think it's the end of the story yet, in terms of Rh genetics.

Weatherall: What's the function of the Rh antigen?

Avent: Some work done by Ann-Marie Marini in Bruno André's lab in Belgium has indicated that they are very closely related to ammonium transporters in lower organisms.[108] There is some direct evidence that they are involved in ammonium transport. Yet other work in the New York Blood Center has shown that Rh protein expression is elevated in response to high CO_2 levels in green algae.[109] So there is some possibility that Rh proteins are involved in CO_2 transport as well as another gas transporter on the surface of red blood cells. The jury's out really, in terms of what the precise functions are. Ammonium transporters may be involved in CO_2 transport, but Rh-null individuals[109a] have deficiencies in all Rh proteins on the surface of their red blood cells, so the function isn't absolutely critical. Clearly there are other proteins in red blood cell membranes that transport CO_2 as well. So there's probably a dual role for Rh proteins at the moment, but the final picture isn't there just yet.

Weatherall: Thanks very much. Any questions or comments about this?

Professor Ian Franklin: Is there any advantage in being rhesus-negative or positive on a population basis? Why is there such a clear polymorphism?

Kumpel: If you are a fetus, maybe it's an advantage to be rhesus-negative, because then your red blood cells can't get destroyed by anti-D. It is not yet known how rhesus-negativity emerged, because it's only in Caucasians that the gene is lacking. There's a pseudogene in Africans. It's really a question for another afternoon I should think, because it's only arisen in whites and not in blacks or Asians.[110]

Avent: I think Belinda is right. The point was initially made by Peter Agre at Johns Hopkins and Jean-Pierre Cartron in Paris. The D-negative phenotype

---

108 Marini *et al.* (1997).

109 Soupene *et al.* (2002).

109a Professor Neil Avent wrote: 'Null individuals are not the same as Rh-negative. They are extremely rare individuals that completely lack Rh proteins from their red cells. They have distinct biochemical anomalies which are not found in RhD-negative individuals.' E-mail to Dr Daphne Christie, 28 September 2004.

110 Daniels (2002): 208–9.

probably did arise as a response to haemolytic disease and the fact that you had a benefit in being rhesus-negative. It has arisen as two different genetic polymorphisms: the Caucasian D gene deletion and the black D-negative phenotype that is due to a mutated Rh-D gene. So there are two separate ways of being D-negative and there are many others that we know of as well. So about 7 per cent is D-negative in black populations and 15 per cent in whites.[111]

Weatherall: This is a kind of general situation with a lot of blood group genetics at the moment. The mechanisms for variation are still, to put it mildly, very speculative, but it's going to be a very interesting story I think. Now to get back to the practicalities. Before I ask the fetal medicine folk to summarize the impact they think all this has made on fetal medicine, could you update us on the management of the prophylaxis over recent years in terms of the role of monoclonal antibodies, source of anti-D material, and so on? Where do we stand at the moment?

Anstee: There has been a programme for more than 15 years to develop and trial monoclonal anti-D as an alternative to the use of polyclonal anti-D. Studies in male volunteers have shown that monoclonal anti-D is effective.[112] This programme is still going on at the Bio Products Laboratory (BPL), Elstree.[112a] But the availability of anti-D from immunized volunteers, as I understand it, is not a problem at the moment, and indeed, the material that's being used in this country is fractionated from plasma, from anti-D donors, purchased from the USA. I think there hasn't been pressure to push the monoclonal antibody product because the availability of the conventional product is not limiting at the moment. There was a period when availability of anti-D in this country was a problem, but that was when we were using our own donor material to provide the product, in a drive for self-sufficiency for such products. However, the decision was made to source plasma from outside the UK (in response to the crisis over variant Creutzfeldt-Jakob disease), and since plasma was being purchased for all products, anti-D could be purchased. So what's happened at the moment, as far as I understand, is that there is no shortage of polyclonal material for fractionation. The cost of bringing the human monoclonal alternative to market is extremely high. The absence of real pressure to provide a product when it is not

---

[111] Colin *et al.* (1991); Singleton *et al.* (2000).

[112] Kumpel *et al.* (1995).

[112a] BPL is one of the UK's largest suppliers of plasma-derived products. It was established by the Lister Institute and has been part of the NHS for over 50 years. See www.sovereign-publications.com/bpl.htm (site visited 1 October 2004).

a problem to source it through the conventional route, has taken the drive away from delivering the monoclonal product. So it's there, and it's going through clinical trials, but it's not available yet.

Tovey: When we had to produce a lot of anti-D from our own resources, this produced a major problem in Britain, because obviously our main source was mothers with antibody, and that was decreasing with the success. There were two procedures that helped us to tackle this problem. First of all was the introduction of plasmapheresis.[113] This meant taking a donation from a donor with high levels of antibody, centrifuging it, removing the plasma and returning the red blood cells to the donor. This was then repeated. Thus, we finished up with two donations of valuable plasma. Later this technique could be performed by a machine, a technique pioneered by my colleague, Dr Angela Robinson.[114]

The second way was deliberately to immunize Rh-negative male volunteers, and this was obviously an ethical dilemma. One was proposing to inject 'foreign' Rh-positive cells into these volunteers, bringing with it the rare but possible transmission of disease (for example, HIV) or the development in these volunteers of other blood group antibodies or white cell antibodies. As I will explain later, we did everything possible to avoid these complications, but we could not guarantee 100 per cent protection. However, in many centres we did succeed in obtaining considerable numbers of male volunteers and, as far as I know, there has been only one case that has caused problems. That was a very unfortunate case where a man, years later, developed renal failure, and unfortunately he couldn't have a kidney transplant because of the white cell antibodies he had developed, obviously most likely as a result of the immunization. The donor red blood cells were chosen from donors who had donated at least 40 times and the patients receiving their blood had suffered no ill effects. The red blood cells did not contain antigens such as little c or Kell, which often cause antibodies to develop, and the cells were washed to remove white cells. So, over a long time, we did our best in Britain in order to raise enough anti-D to allow not only post-delivery prevention, but also antenatal prevention. But I think it should be recorded that over this long period of time, a considerable number of Rh-negative men, in spite of the possible complications, were prepared to be injected with a foreign substance, in order to help Rh-negative women – truly altruistic acts, as they received no payment.

---

[113] See, for example, Graham-Pole (1975); Fraser *et al.* (1976).

[114] Robinson *et al.* (1983).

Franklin: It is just worth pointing out that in the USA the reason they have no problem getting their supplies is that they pay donors the going rate. I have to say as a clinician I think it is unfortunate that there hasn't been a move towards a successful monoclonal antibody. One other interesting point about, I think it was Ronnie Finn, who changed the formulation to avoid serum hepatitis.[115] I suppose there are always going to be question marks over allogeneic blood-derived products, and I think a monoclonal product would be infinitely preferable, as far as I am concerned.

Dr Angela Robinson: I would like to comment on the development in the clinical trials of the monoclonal antibody. Last week I was at the Bio Products Laboratory where they were telling us about these trials with a recombinant monoclonal antibody. The big difficulty is that the times are so different. Imagine the size of the study that would be required to get it through the European Committee for Proprietary Medicinal Products (CPMP),[116] which is the European regulatory committee, and the ethical problems of using this unknown substance in pregnant women. You couldn't choose a more difficult trial to undertake. The numbers that they want, to give the study sufficient statistical power to prove effectiveness, are just so huge. It's almost certainly beyond BPL's ability to fund without some collaboration with a huge commercial partner. It's very sad that the times are such that where you could have done this study in Finn's day, it's proving almost impossible to do it today.

Mr Ian MacKenzie: There is, however, a need to develop a recombinant monoclonal product because, in today's climate, patients want to know the risks they might be letting themselves in for, and with the recent NICE (National Institute for Clinical Excellence) guidelines, all non-sensitized rhesus-negative women should be offered antenatal prophylaxis.[117] I know from experience of

---

[115] See page 29.

[116] The Committee for Proprietary Medicinal Products is the scientific committee of the European Agency for the Evaluation of Medicinal Products (EMEA). For further details visit www.mca.gov.uk/ourwork/licensingmeds/european/europelic.htm (site visited 16 September 2004).

[117] National Institute for Clinical Excellence (NICE) (2002). Dr Christopher Everett wrote: 'The Edinburgh Consensus Conference on anti-D prophylaxis, 7 and 8 April 1997, gave their unanimous support for the introduction of antenatal prophylaxis, already standard practice in other countries [see Urbaniak (1998a, 1998b)]. However, there followed considerable opposition and unnecessary delay from the Royal College of Obstetricians and Gynaecologists, London, associated with extreme reluctance from the College of Midwives and the UK Central Council for Nursing, Midwifery and Health Visiting (UKCC) to support the recommendations. As a result the whole issue had to be referred to NICE in order to resolve the impasse with yet more delay, and fetal morbidity!' Letter to Mrs Wendy Kutner, 7 June 2003.

trying to recruit women to trials, they are very reluctant to take part in a study that involves a blood product, because of the risks that exist. So there is a very big drive to develop a recombinant monoclonal product.

Dr Edwin Massey: It's interesting. At huge cost, the haemophilic treatment in the UK has changed in the last few years.[118] In Wales, a recombinant factor VIII and factor IX have taken over completely from human plasma-derived factors. The same is now being undertaken in England. You would have thought that there would be a strong impetus to be doing the same for pregnant women with anti-D.

Kumpel: I would like to say that we all know how effective the polyclonal product is, and it has been proved to be extremely safe by nearly all the manufacturers. There's no reason why the monoclonal shouldn't be so as well, and you understand the concerns of the regulatory authorities in producing a medicine for healthy women during and after pregnancy. The only worry that I would have is that most of the European countries and some of the smaller countries don't manufacture their own anti-D because of the expense, so that most of it is now purchased from North American sources. If there was any compromising of the supply from North America, either a new virus or something or another factor that reduces the supply, then there is nothing in the pipeline as a reserve. The monoclonal is not yet ready and most other countries can't come up with their own. If there's not enough antibody, we know we will be back to the situation in the 1960s where there will be deaths from haemolytic disease, well, possibly not deaths, but it will be a severe problem for the obstetricians and I think it's a shame that the regulatory authorities do have to be so stringent in producing an alternative supply.

Finn: May I mention something that is highly speculative? At the very beginning we decided purely empirically to pool our sera together. I don't know any scientific reason for this but, empirically, if you mix them all together you are going to get a broader antigenic coverage. My understanding is that a monoclonal antibody has been tried in experimental circumstances and found not to be very effective. What I am going to suggest is that if you do eventually make monoclonal antibodies, they should be mixed together afterwards and not simply rely on a single monoclonal. I don't know whether that is nonsense, but it's just a thought I've had.

---

[118] See Tansey and Christie (1999): 35, 75–7.

Anstee: Just a point to clarify that the monoclonal product that's been developed at the Bio Products Laboratory is a mixture of two monoclonal antibodies. So it's not just a one shot. Although I think there is some evidence that if you have the right antibody one will work. To make a product comprising a large number of different monoclonal antibodies would add greatly to the cost of the development programme.

Weatherall: I think we have given that enough fresh air. All medical advances produce another set of problems, but they don't sound insurmountable. We should ask Timos Valaes and Charles Rodeck if they would like to say a few words on the total impact of this on fetal medicine. Somebody asked me in the interval if you could mention phototherapy along the way, because it's something that we have neglected a bit this afternoon. It is the one form of treatment that we haven't explored.

Valaes: The impact, as far as the neonate, was completed by the mid-1970s. By that time, almost all babies born alive and not extremely immature or hydropic would survive intact. Phototherapy helped in reducing the number of exchange transfusions necessary to keep serum bilirubin at a safe level.[119] From our vista as neonatologists, we saw the whole battlefield being transferred from treatment of the neonate to *in utero* interventions to improve the chances for survival of the fetus. As I said before, these efforts were evolving against the backdrop of diminishing numbers of isoimmunized pregnant women as the result of the preventive programmes. At the same time, neonatology and fetal medicine have exploded in their techniques to take on other big problems. I don't think we are going to see many isoimmunized women. Seldom there will be lapses in the preventive programmes or failures of anti-D globulin prevention because of a large feto-maternal transfusion that was not detected and the dose of anti-D was not adjusted accordingly.

Rodeck: That's not quite our experience. There has, of course, been a major reduction in the incidence and prevalence of women with antibodies, but we still have, as do most fetal medicine units, a couple of women on the go at any time with antibodies, and we would still be doing about 30 transfusions a year. These are on average a couple a month, which means there is a serious risk that this will lead to more operators becoming deskilled. But we have left the story I think, with Liley's intraperitoneal transfusion, and of course that didn't help

[119] Dr Christopher Everett wrote: 'As a GP doing midwifery, phototherapy was a most helpful and significant treatment in reducing bilirubin levels in a maternity unit away from a general hospital.' Letter to Mrs Wendy Kutner, 7 June 2003.

the very early, very severely affected fetus that was hydropic because of poor absorption of the transfused blood. Liley was given the idea by a paediatrician from Africa, who had gone through his unit, who said that's how they transfused their sickle cell children. The basis of this transfusion is that it gets absorbed from the peritoneal cavity into the lymphatics and then up the thoracic duct and into the circulation. Hydropic fetuses don't absorb this, so that you have the paradox of the most severely affected fetuses not actually benefiting from that treatment. In the 1970s a whole variety of techniques were coming together, which enabled and increased activity in intrauterine intervention, and there was a lot of interest in fetal blood sampling and that was partly the fault of our chairman, Professor Weatherall, who devised a technique for the diagnosis of haemoglobinopathies, and so a lot of us were interested in that area. Humphry Ward and Ian MacKenzie, in this room, were involved in that too. At that time, at King's College Hospital, London, we were developing a fetoscopic method for obtaining fetal blood, which resulted in pure samples from the umbilical cord, and if you could take out blood from the cord, it meant you could put in transfused blood as well.

But our problem was that we couldn't get hold of any rhesus patients. They were all at the Rhesus Centre at Lewisham Hospital and were guarded jealously. I happened to be in Oxford giving a talk and returned on the train to London with David Whitmore, who was a haematologist from Lewisham (he was part of their impressive multidisciplinary group). I said to him, 'This is a blood disease, wouldn't you like to get fetal blood?' He liked the idea and invited me to give a talk there, and that's how we set up a collaboration. The first patient they referred for our first intravascular transfusion had five antibodies with astronomically high titres and the most horrendously hydropic fetus. These hydropic fetuses are in heart failure. To give a blood transfusion directly into the fetal circulation was of great concern because there was the risk of worsening the heart failure and causing fetal death. In fact, it's quite remarkable the amount of blood that a fetus will tolerate: you can increase its feto-placental blood volume by 200 per cent, it will survive. Anyway, this fetus survived, so we got a steady stream of the most severe patients from Lewisham. They kept the less severe ones for themselves. We published our earliest experience in the *Lancet* in 1981.[120]

The fetoscopic technique was actually technically very difficult and then by the mid-1980s Fernand Daffos in Paris had devised an ultrasound-guided

[120] Rodeck *et al.* (1981).

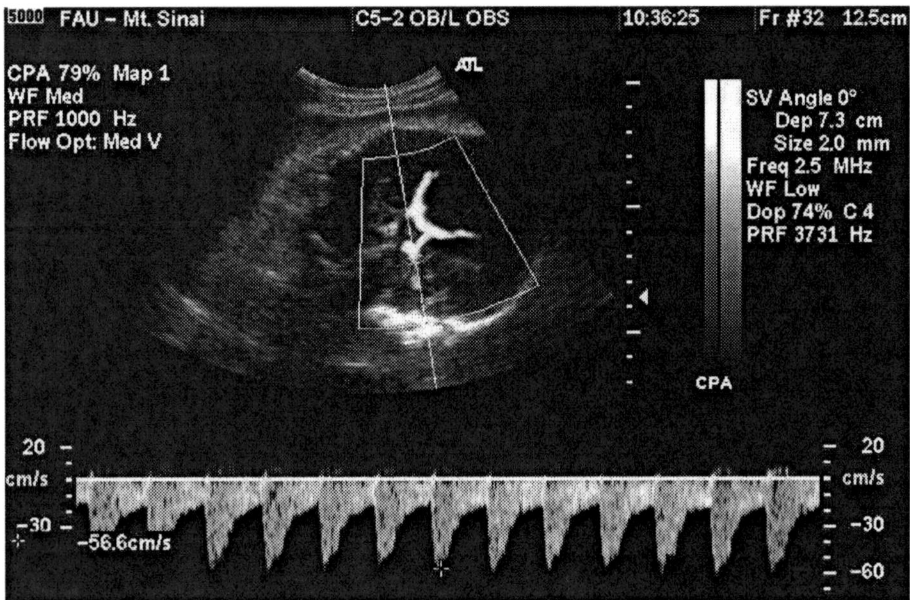

Figure 6: Non-invasive assessment of fetal anaemia by measurement of velocity of fetal blood in the fetal middle cerebral artery. Top: Doppler image of the fetal head showing the Circle of Willis with the Doppler gate on the distal middle cerebral artery. Bottom: Doppler wave derived from the middle cerebral artery showing a peak systolic velocity of 56.6 cms^{-1}.

needling technique of the umbilical cord which was much easier and this became much more widespread.[121] It was taken up in many different parts of the world, and it led to a rise in further investigation, and treatment. One could say that it was during this time that fetal medicine was emerging as a discipline, but it was very much a diagnostic rather than a therapeutic activity, and the rhesus model gave us an opportunity to develop a therapeutic arm. Intravascular transfusion was highly successful, and it was most gratifying how, over and over again, we saw hydropic fetuses in which the hydrops disappeared and babies were delivered at quite late gestation in very good condition. Because they all had O-negative blood in their circulation and their own erythropoeisis had been switched off, they got very little jaundice so that exchange transfusion almost disappeared. There are fewer and fewer patients now needing *in utero* transfusions so we do have problems with maintaining those skills. On the other hand, the whole area has become much less invasive than it was. For example, amniocentesis is now no longer needed to assess

[121] Daffos *et al.* (1983).

severity. We use Doppler ultrasound to investigate the velocity of blood in the fetal circulation, particularly in the middle cerebral artery (Figure 6), which is inversely proportional to the haemoglobin level.[122] Anaemic fetuses have higher velocities at which the blood moves, and so we can assess roughly their degree of anaemia, and then can proceed to blood transfusion, on the basis of this non-invasive test.[123]

The other very useful recent development is the discovery of free fetal DNA in maternal blood. That was based on an observation in cancer patients that they had free DNA in their blood, and then Dennis Lo, in Oxford and now in Hong Kong, found fetal DNA in maternal plasma.[124] This means that one can detect paternally-inherited genes in the maternal blood. So the fetus of a rhesus-negative woman can be genotyped from her blood, an advance that Neil Avent has been involved in as well and on which we have collaborated. Now that we can genotype the fetus in a much less invasive way, we need something to block the antigen/antibody interaction, so that we can treat the fetus without having to resort to transfusion.

Weatherall: Thanks. That was a very stimulating talk. You mean you actually measure the haemoglobin level in the fetus relatively accurately on the speed of circulation by ultrasound?

Rodeck: We know the normal range of velocities in the fetal middle cerebral artery, and if the fetal blood velocity is higher than that, then there is a 90–95 per cent chance that it is anaemic.

Weatherall: How accurate is this?

Rodeck: The detection or the sensitivity is in the region of 90 per cent that the haemoglobin is below 7g/dl.[125]

---

[122] Mari *et al.* (2000).

[123] Dr Sheila Duncan wrote: 'In the early 1970s when prophylaxis came in there is an impression that the disorder disappeared. The cohort of women already immunized in the 1960s, if young, went on having babies for many years and were supplemented by a steady stream of women whose prophylaxis failed or who were immunized during pregnancy or came from overseas. Obstetricians still had to treat the established condition, in the 1960s and 1970s by intraperitoneal transfusion. In the late 1970s and early 1980s plasmapheresis of severe cases was tried in an attempt to avoid the hazards of fetal invasive procedures. An important stimulus for this was the development of intensive neonatal care [see Christie and Tansey (2001)] so that delivery from about 28 weeks could be considered.' From a letter to Dr Daphne Christie, 19 November 2003.

[124] Lo (2001).

[125] Mari *et al.* (2000).

Weatherall: So there have been extraordinary advances and I suppose you would argue, historically, that quite a number of them were pushed along by the rhesus problem.

Rodeck: Yes, indeed. In any case, I think that Liley's work, both diagnostic and therapeutic, is a beacon and was way, way ahead of his time. I suppose all of us have been catching up a bit with the benefit of much better technology. First of all, the use of ultrasound has enabled invasive procedures to be much safer, they would be impossible without it, and of course it also now allows us to avoid some invasive procedures.[126]

Valaes: Going back to the basics, I would like to stress the importance of being able to evaluate with reliable antibody tests, like the Coombs test, the presence of isoimmune haemolytic disease of the newborn. This cleared the field and enabled us to start looking for other causes of severe neonatal jaundice and kernicterus – causes like G6PD (glucose 6-phosphate dehydrogenase) deficiency which in many parts of the world plays as important a role as Rh incompatibility used to play before effective prevention of isoimmunization.[127] Without these tests, we would be still talking about rare antibodies and unknown blood group antigens to explain these cases.

Robinson: I would like to ask Charles Rodeck a question. How early now can you, or would you reckon, to safely do a direct intrauterine transfusion?

Rodeck: We try to avoid it before 20 weeks, because the risks are higher, but for fetuses that are hydropic at 18 weeks, you have to do something about it and you can do an intravascular transfusion.

Hunter: I would like to make two points. The first is about the economic and institutional factors that changed dramatically during Cyril Clarke's professional life. From 1936 to 1939, he had a life insurance practice at Grocer's Hall in London, EC2, in order to earn his living. With the inception of the National Health Service in 1948, he had a salary and this gave him a degree of freedom with which he could pursue original research that has been discussed today.

Secondly, I would like to mention that in his presidential address to the Liverpool Medical Institution in 1970, he spoke about how his original interest

---

[126] This was the subject of a previous Witness Seminar, 'Looking at the Unborn: Historical aspects of obstetric ultrasound'. See Tansey and Christie (2000).

[127] For a review see Clarke (1972).

in inheritance of rhesus blood groups arose from his study of inheritance in butterflies. His address had the title 'The Deceptive Way of Life'.[128]

MacKenzie: Can we mention one other development that has had a very significant impact upon obstetric practice and neonatal practice, and that is the introduction of routine antenatal anti-D prophylaxis, which as far as I recall was introduced initially in the 1970s in Canada by Bowman,[129] and Derrick Tovey[130] promoted it here in the early 1980s?[131] It's now almost a statutory requirement that we provide it for all pregnant rhesus-negative women, although at the moment I don't think most units are managing to do that. But the impact that we have noticed in Oxford since 1986, when we introduced routine antenatal prophylaxis for all nulliparous rhesus-negative women, has been considerable. In the 1980s we would see round about ten women a year in our district, with rhesus D isoimmunization among 5000–6000 women delivering a year; that proportion of women would be expected with routine postnatal delivery prophylaxis, with prophylaxis for other precipitating and potentially sensitizing events during the antenatal period. The figure of sensitized pregnancies is now down to zero or one per year, as a result of giving routine antenatal prophylaxis as well as the routine postnatal prophylaxis to all nulliparous rhesus-negative women. In other words, we have almost eliminated anti-D isoimmunization in our population. I think it now works out, when we did our analysis, that there is a 0.3 per cent incidence. Some cases will always slip through, but I think that does mean, as Professor Rodeck says, that the number of severely affected cases will diminish throughout the country, and there probably should only be one or two centres in the UK that will be treating these severely compromised rhesus pregnancies.

Tovey: There was a major drop in the incidence of anti-D following the introduction of postnatal anti-D, but from 1975 to 1980 it levelled out,[132] and the incidence of sensitization altered very little over the next few years. This was primarily due to the fact that there are mothers who were developing antibodies before delivery. In other words, it was too late for the postnatal anti-D, and that's why antenatal prophylaxis was introduced, first of all, by John

[128] Clarke (1970): 4; Weatherall (2002).

[129] Bowman *et al.* (1978).

[130] Tovey *et al.* (1983).

[131] For a history, see Wegmann and Gluck (1996).

[132] See Figure 5, page 23.

Bowman in Canada.[133] The other point is this: when the antibody sensitization dropped by 70 per cent over that period of time, the death rate of babies dropped 96 per cent, which showed that not only were anti-D injections helpful but there was a great improvement in the babies' antenatal and postnatal care. It wasn't only the anti-D injections. We were very successful at saving babies' lives, but not quite so successful at preventing mothers becoming sensitized. Therefore, in order to try to do that, we introduced antenatal prophylaxis in this country, as you know. The work we reported in the Yorkshire trial did show one thing: it was very important to give antenatal prophylaxis in the first pregnancy.[134] We did not consider it necessary to give anti-D during every pregnancy, for example, to a woman in her eighth. You can reduce the mortality considerably by simply just giving it in the first rhesus-positive pregnancy.

Robinson: I want to make a comment, sitting next to this very modest man, that Dr Derrick Tovey did the first proper antenatal prophylaxis trials.[135] Twenty years ago he started it, and 20 years on they have now decided nationally that it's a good thing to do. That very early work was done by Derrick in the Yorkshire trials.

Tovey: Another point to add. It was done for 2000 mothers and 2000 pregnancies, and we didn't get a penny in any way. We did it entirely on our own money!

Dr Mahes de Silva: I wonder if I could ask a question of Professor Rodeck? There have been reports of intravenous immunoglobulin being effective for the treatment of very severe Rh disease,[136] and with cases getting fewer, has the need for intervention by transfusion become less?

Rodeck: Yes, there are no randomized trials of high dose IV Ig (intravenous immunoglobulin) infusions, whether they are given into the mother or indeed given to the fetus, and personally I have some scepticism that it works for that particular antigen–antibody interaction. It seems to be of some value for autoimmune thrombocytopaenia, but again I don't think there are any randomized studies that demonstrate that either.

Weatherall: I would like to thank you for being such a great audience and taking part so well, and making a chairman's job so easy. This has been a marvellous story. I don't know what the lessons are, except that there was some

---

[133] Bowman *et al.* (1978).

[134] Tovey *et al.* (1983).

[135] Tovey *et al.* (1983).

[136] See, for example, Greenough (2001).

excellent science leading up to it, and then a very unusual man in Liverpool who was a bit of a polymath with a tremendous flair for picking out bright young people, as you have seen this afternoon. It seems to me that the concept of building up a group of young people round such a person, and not pushing too hard in which direction they go, letting them follow their noses, has proved a wonderful success in this case. So, although that may not be a message of enormous help to the government or our health research supporting bodies, that's what real life is about, and it's been a fantastic story. I would like to congratulate everybody in the field, not just the Liverpool team, but also the people who have made it possible by the early strategic build up. I'd also like to thank the Wellcome Trust, and the History of Twentieth Century Medicine Group for bringing us here this afternoon.

References

Aidin R, Corner B D, Tovey G. (1950) Kernicterus and prematurity. *Lancet* **i**: 1153–4.

Aird I, Bentall H H, Fraser-Roberts J A. (1953) A relationship between cancer of the stomach and the ABO blood groups. *British Medical Journal* **i**: 799–801.

Aird I, Bentall H H, Mehigan J A, Roberts J A F. (1954) The blood groups in relation to peptic ulceration and carcinoma of the colon, rectum, breast and bronchus: An association between the ABO groups and peptic ulceration. *British Medical Journal* **ii**: 315–21.

Altmann P, Bruce J E, Karnicki J. (1975a) The influence of intrauterine transfusion upon birth weight in rhesus haemolytic disease. *European Journal of Obstetrics, Gynecology, and Reproductive Biology* **5**: 247–50.

Altmann P, Bruce J E, Karnicki J. (1975b) Blood in amniotic fluid following intrauterine transfusion and its effect on premature onset of labor. *Journal of Perinatal Medicine* **3**: 166–71.

Anon. (1957) Sir Lionel Whitby (1895–1956). *Annals of the Royal College of Surgeons of England* **20**:134–7.

Anon. (1960) Medical Societies: Liverpool Medical Institution, Erythroblastosis. *Lancet* **i**: 526.

Anon. (1968) Sir Lionel Ernest Howard Whitby. *Munk's Roll* **5**: 444–5.

Anon. (1971) Alistair Livingston Gunn. *The Journal of Obstetrics and Gynaecology of the British Commonwealth* **78**: 190–1.

Armitage P, Mollison P L. (1953) Further analysis of controlled trials of treatment of haemolytic disease of the newborn. *Journal of Obstetrics and Gynaecology* **60**: 605–20.

Avent N D, Ridgwell K, Tanner M J, Anstee D J. (1990) cDNA cloning of a 30 kDa erythrocyte membrane protein associated with Rh (rhesus)-blood-group-antigen expression. *Biochemical Journal* **271**: 821–5.

Ballantyne J W. (1892) *The Diseases and Deformities of the Foetus.* Edinburgh: Oliver & Boyd, Ltd.

Bangham D R, Kirkwood T B, Wybrow G, Hughes-Jones N C, Gunson H H. (1978) International collaborative study of assay of anti-D (anti-Rh_o) immunoglobulin. *British Journal of Haematology* **38**: 407–23.

Bangham D R. (2000) *A History of Biological Standardisation: The Characterization and Measurement of Complex Molecules Important in Clinical and Research Medicine: Contributions from the UK 1900–95: What, Why, How, Where and by Whom – A Personal Account.* London: The Society for Endocrinology.

Bernstein F. (1924) Ergebnissse einer biostatistischen zusammem-fassenden betrachtung über die erblichen blutstrukturen des menschen. *Klinische Wochenschrift* **3**: 1495–7.

Berriman D A. (1971) The Rhesus Unit at Lewisham. 3. *Midwives Chronicle* **85**: 336–8.

Bevis D C. (1950) Composition of liquor amnii in haemolytic disease of the newborn. *Lancet* **ii**: 443.

Bevis D C. (1952) The antenatal prediction of haemolytic disease of the newborn. *Lancet* **i**: 395–8.

Bevis D C. (1956) Blood pigments in haemolytic disease of the newborn. *Journal of Obstetrics and Gynaecology of the British Empire* **63**: 68–75.

Bodmer W F. (1992) Early British discoveries in human genetics: Contributions of R A Fisher and J B S Haldane to the development of blood groups. *American Journal of Human Genetics* **50**: 671–6.

Bordet J, Gay F P. (1906) Sur les relations des sensibilisatrices avec l'alexine. *Annales de l'Institut Pasteur* **20**: 467–98.

Bordet J, Streng O. (1909) Les phénomènes d'adsorption de la conglutinine du sérum de boeuf. *Annales de l'Institut Pasteur* **49**: 260–76.

Bowman J M, Chown B, Lewis M, Pollock J M. (1978) Rh-isoimmunisation during pregnancy: Antenatal prophylaxis. *Canadian Medical Association Journal* **118:** 623–7.

Buchanan J A, Higley E T. (1921) The relationship of blood groups to disease. *British Journal of Experimental Pathology* **2**: 247–55.

Cherif-Zahar B, Bloy C, Le Van Kim C, Blanchard D, Bailly P, Hermand P, Salmon C, Cartron J P, Colin Y. (1990) Molecular cloning and protein structure of a human blood group Rh polypeptide. *Proceedings of the National Academy of Sciences* **87**: 6243–7.

Christie D A, Tansey E M. (2001) Origins of Neonatal Intensive Care in the UK. *Wellcome Witnesses to Twentieth Century Medicine.* Volume 9. London: The Wellcome Trust Centre for the History of Medicine at UCL.

Clarke C A. (1968) The prevention of 'Rhesus' babies. *Scientific American* **219**: 46–52.

Clarke C. (1970) The deceptive way of life. *Transactions and Reports of the Liverpool Medical Institution*, 4.

Clarke C A. (1972) Prevention of Rh isoimmunization. *Progress in Medical Genetics* **8**: 169–223.

Clarke C A. (1977) Philip Macdonald Sheppard. *Biographical Memoirs of Fellows of the Royal Society* **23**: 465–500.

Clarke C A. (1985) Robert Russell Race. *Biographical Memoirs of Fellows of the Royal Society* **31**: 455–92.

Clarke C A. (1990) Professor Sir Ronald Fisher. *British Medical Journal* **301**: 1446–8.

Clarke C A, Finn R. (1977) Prevention of Rh haemolytic disease: Background of the Liverpool work. *American Journal of Obstetrics and Gynecology* **127**: 538–9.

Clarke C A, Mollison P L. (1989) Deaths from Rh haemolytic disease of the fetus and newborn 1977–87. *Journal of the Royal College of Physicians* **23**: 181–4.

Clarke C, Hussey R M. (1994) Decline in deaths from rhesus haemolytic disease of the newborn. *Journal of the Royal College of Physicians* **28**: 310–1.

Clarke C A, Finn R, Lehane D, McConnell R B, Sheppard P M, Woodrow J C. (1966) Dose of anti-D gamma-globulin in prevention of Rh-haemolytic disease of the newborn. *British Medical Journal* **ii**: 213–4.

Clarke C A, Sheppard P M, Thornton I W B. (1968) The genetics of the mimetic butterfly *Papilio memnon. Philosophical Transactions of the Royal Society B* **254**: 37–89.

Colin Y, Chérif-Zahar B, Le Van Kim C, Raynal V, Van Huffel V, Cartron J P. (1991) Genetic basis of the RhD-positive and RhD-negative blood group polymorphism as determined by Southern analysis. *Blood* **78**: 2747–52.

Combined study. (1966) Prevention of Rh-haemolytic disease: Results of the clinical trial. A combined study from centres in England and Baltimore. *British Medical Journal* **ii**: 907–14.

Coombs F H C, Mourant A, Race R R. (1945a) Detection of weak and 'incomplete' Rh agglutinins: A new test. *Lancet* **ii**: 15.

Coombs F H C, Mourant A, Race R R. (1945b) A new test for the detection of weak and 'incomplete Rh agglutinins'. *British Journal of Experimental Pathology* **26**: 255–66.

Corner B D. (1947) The rhesus factors II: Haemolytic disease of the newborn. *Bristol Medico-Chirurgical Journal* **64**: 72–90.

Corner B D. (1958) Hyperbilirubinaemia in premature infants treated by exchange blood transfusion. *Proceedings of the Royal Society of Medicine* **51**: 1019–22.

Craft A W. (2004) Walker, William. *Munk's Roll* **11**. See www.rcplondon.ac.uk/scripts/munk_details.asp?ID=4586 (site visited 27 October 2004).

Crow J F. (1993) Felix Bernstein and the first human marker locus. *Genetics* **133**: 4–7.

Daffos F, Capella-Pavlovsky M, Forestier F. (1983) Fetal blood sampling via the umbilical cord using a needle guided by ultrasound. Report of 66 cases. *Prenatal Diagnosis* **3**: 271–7.

Daniels G. (2002) *Human Blood Groups.* 2nd edn. Oxford: Blackwell Science.

Davidsohn I, Masaitis L, Stern K. (1956) Experimental studies on Rh immunization. *American Journal of Clinical Pathology* **26**: 833–43.

Diamond L K. (1947) Erythroblastosis foetalis. *Proceedings of the Royal Society of Medicine B* **40**: 546–50.

Diamond L K. (1948) Replacement transfusion as a treatment for erythroblastosis fetalis. *Pediatrics* **2**: 520–4.

Diamond L K. (1980a) A tribute to Dr Philip Levine. *American Journal of Clinical Pathology* **74**: 368–70.

Diamond L K. (1980b) The story of our blood groups, in Wintrobe M M. (ed.) *Blood, Pure and Eloquent.* Chapter 20. New York: McGraw-Hill Book Company, 691–717.

Diamond L K. (1983) Historic perspective on 'exchange transfusion'. *Vox Sanguinis* **45**: 333–5.

Diamond L K, Denton R L. (1945) Rh agglutination in various media with particular reference to the value of albumin. *Journal of Laboratory and Clinical Medicine* **30**: 821.

Diamond L K, Allen F H Jr, Thomas W O Jr. (1951) Erythroblastosis fetalis. VII. Treatment with exchange transfusion. *New England Journal of Medicine* **244**: 39–49.

Dodsworth H. (1996) Blood transfusion services in the UK. *Journal of the Royal College of Physicians of London* **30**: 457–64.

Elson C J, Woodrow J C, Donohoe W T. (1971) Clearance of erythrocytes and the immune response. *Vox Sanguinis* **20**: 201–8.

Finn R, Clarke C A, Donohoe W T, McConnell R B, Sheppard P M, Lehane D, Kulke W. (1961) Experimental studies on the prevention of Rh haemolytic disease. *British Medical Journal* **i**: 1486–90.

Fisher R A. (1947) The Rhesus factor: A study in scientific method. *American Scientist* **35**: 95–103.

Ford E B. (1945) Polymorphism. *Biological Reviews* **20**: 73–88.

Fraser I. (2002) Geoffrey Harold Tovey. *Transfusion Medicine* **12**: 151–2.

Fraser I D, Bothamley J A, Bennett M O, Airth G R, Lehane D, McCarthy M, Roberts F M. (1976) Intensive antenatal plasmapheresis in severe rhesus isoimmunisation. *Lancet* **i**: 6–9.

Freda V J, Gorman J G, Pollack W. (1964) Successful prevention of experimental Rh sensitization in man with an anti-Rh gamma2-globulin antibody preparation. *Transfusion* 77: 26–32.

Freda V J, Gorman J G, Pollack W. (1977) Prevention of Rh-hemolytic disease with Rh-immune globulin. *American Journal of Obstetrics and Gynecology* **1278**: 456–60.

Freed D L J. (2004) Obituary. Ronald Finn. *British Medical Journal* **328**: 1501.

Gahmberg C G. (1982) Molecular identification of the human Rh_o (D) antigen. *FEBS Letters* **140**: 93–7.

Giangrande P L. (2000) The history of blood transfusion. Historical review. *British Journal of Haematology* **110**: 758–67.

Giblett E R. (1994) Philip Levine. *Biographical Memoirs of the National Academy of Sciences* **63**: 323–47.

Graham-Pole J. (1975) Proceedings: Plasmapheresis in rhesus disease. *Scottish Medical Journal* **20**: 168–9.

Greenough A. (2001) The role of immunoglobulins in neonatal Rhesus haemolytic disease. *BioDrugs* **15**: 533–41.

Gridwood R H. (1990) Fifty years of an organized blood transfusion service in Scotland. *Scottish Medical Journal* **35**: 24–8.

Gunson H H, Dodsworth H. (1996) Fifty years of blood transfusion. *Transfusion Medicine* **6**: 1–88.

Harper P S. (1995) Genetic testing, common diseases and health service provision. *Lancet* **346**: 1645–6.

Heyman B, Wigzell H. (1984) Immunoregulation by monoclonal sheep erythrocyte-specific IgG antibodies: Suppression is correlated to level of antigen binding and not to isotype. *Journal of Immunology* **132**: 1136–43.

Hughes-Jones N C. (1967) The estimation of the concentration and the equilibrium constant of anti-D. *Immunology* **12**: 565–71.

Hughes-Jones N, Tippett P. (2003) Ruth Ann Sanger. *Biographical Memoirs of Fellows of the Royal Society* **49**: 461–73.

Karlsson M C, Wernersson S, Diaz de Stahl T, Gustavsson S, Heyman B. (1999) Efficient IgG-mediated suppression of primary antibody responses in Fc gamma receptor-deficient mice. *Proceedings of the National Academy of Sciences* **96**: 2244–9.

Kevles D J. (1995) *In the Name of Eugenics.* Cambridge, MA: Harvard University Press.

Kleihauer E, Braun H, Betke K. (1957) Demonstration of fetal hemoglobin in erythrocytes of a blood smear. *Klinische Wochenschrift* **35**: 637–8.

Kumpel B M, Elson C J. (2001) Mechanism of anti-D-mediated immune suppression – a paradox awaiting resolution? *Trends in Immunology* **22**: 26–31.

Kumpel B M, Goodrick M J, Pamphilon D H, Fraser I D, Poole G D, Morse C, Standen G R, Chapman G E, Thomas D P, Anstee D J. (1995) Human Rh D monoclonal antibodies (BRAD-3 and BRAD-5) cause accelerated clearance of Rh D+ red blood cells and suppression of Rh D- immunization in volunteers. *Blood* **86**: 1701–9.

Landsteiner K. (1900) Zur Kenntnis der antifermentativen, lytischen und agglutinierenden wirkungen des blutserums und der lymphe. *Centralblatt für Bakteriologie, Parasitenkunde und Infektionskrankheiten* **27**: 357–62.

Landsteiner K. (1901) Über agglutinationserscheinungen normalen menschlichen blutes. *Wiener Klinische Wochenschrift* **14**: 1132–4.

Landsteiner K. (1903) Über Beziehungen zwischen dem blutserum und der korperzellen. *Münchener Medizinische Wochenschrift* **50**: 1812–4.

Landsteiner K, Wiener A S. (1940) An agglutination factor in human blood recognized by immune sera for rhesus blood. *Proceedings of the Society for Experimental Biology and Medicine* **43**: 223–9.

Lathe G H. (1955) Exchange transfusion as a means of removing bilirubin in haemolytic disease of the newborn. *British Medical Journal* **i**: 192–6.

Lathe G H, Claireaux A E, Norman A P. (1958) Jaundice in the newborn, in Gairdner D. (ed.) *Recent Advances in Paediatrics.* 2nd edn. London: J & A Churchill Ltd, 87–124, 125–44.

Leggat H M, Gibson J M, Barron S L, Reid M M. (1991) Anti-Kell in pregnancy. *British Journal of Obstetrics and Gynaecology* **98**: 162–5.

Levine P. (1943) Serological factors as possible causes in spontaneous abortions. *Journal of Heredity* **34**: 71–80.

Levine P. (1984) The discovery of Rh haemolytic disease. *Vox Sanguinis* **47**: 187–90.

Levine P, Stetson R. (1939) An unusual case of intra-group agglutination. *Journal of the American Medical Association* **113**: 126–7.

Levine P, Burnham L, Katzin E M, Vogel P. (1941) The role of isoimmunization in the pathogenesis of erythroblastosis fetalis. *American Journal of Obstetrics and Gynecology* **42**: 925–41.

Liley A W. (1961) Liquor amnii analysis in the management of the pregnancy complicated by rhesus sensitization. *American Journal of Obstetrics and Gynecology* **82**: 1359–70.

Liley A W. (1963) Intrauterine transfusion of foetus in haemolytic disease. *British Medical Journal* **ii**: 1107–9.

Lo Y M. (2001) Fetal DNA in maternal plasma: Application to non-invasive blood group genotyping of the fetus. *Transfusion Clinique et Biologique* **8**: 306–10.

Longo L D. (1977) Classic pages in obstetrics and gynecology. Experimental studies on the prevention of Rh haemolytic disease: Ronald Finn, Cyril Astley Clarke, William Thomas Atkin Donohoe, Richard Bonar McConnell, Philip Macdonald Sheppard, Dermot Lehane, and William Kulke. *American Journal of Obstetrics and Gynecology* **127**: 537.

Mari G, Deter R L, Carpenter R L, Rahman F, Zimmerman R, Moise K J Jr, Dorman K F, Ludomirsky A, Gonzalez R, Gomez R, Oz U, Detti L, Copel J A, Bahado-Singh R, Berry S, Martinez-Poyer J, Blackwell S C. (2000) Noninvasive diagnosis by Doppler ultrasonography of fetal anemia due to maternal red-cell alloimmunization. Collaborative Group for Doppler Assessment of the Blood Velocity in Anemic Fetuses. *New England Journal of Medicine* **342**: 9–14.

Marini A-M, Urrestarazu A, Beauwens R, André B. (1997) The Rh (rhesus) blood group polypeptides are related to NH_4^+ transporters. *Trends in Biochemical Sciences* **22**: 460–1.

McCall A J, Holdsworth S. (1945) Haemolytic disease of the newborn caused by the antibody St. *Nature* **155**: 788.

Misson G P, Bishop A C, Watkins W M. (1999) Arthur Ernest Mourant. *Biographical Memoirs of Fellows of the Royal Society* **45**: 331–48.

Mollison P L. (1970) The effect of isoantibodies on red-cell survival. *Annals of the New York Academy of Sciences* **169**: 199–216.

Mollison P L. (2002) Ruth Sanger. *Transfusion* **42**: 125–6.

Mollison P L, Cutbush M. (1951) A method of measuring the severity of a series of cases of haemolytic disease of the newborn. *Blood* **6**: 777–88.

Mollison P L, Cutbush M. (1954) Haemolytic disease of the newborn, in Gairdner D. (ed.) *Recent Advances in Paediatrics*. London: J and A Churchill, 110–32.

Mollison P L, Walker W. (1952) Controlled trials of the treatment of haemolytic disease of the newborn. *Lancet* **i**: 429–33.

Moor-Jankowski J. (1978) Dr Alexander S Wiener 1907–76. *Vox Sanguinis* **34**: 189–90.

Moreschi C. (1908) Neue tatsachen uber die blutkorperchenagglutination. *Zentralblatt für Bakteriologie* **46**: 49–51.

Morgan W T J, Watkins W M. (2000) Unravelling the biochemical basis of blood group ABO and Lewis antigenic specificity. *Glycoconjugate Journal* **17**: 501–30.

Morton J A, Pickles M M. (1947) Use of trypsin in the detection of incomplete anti-Rh antibodies. *Nature* **159**: 779–80.

Mourant A E. (1983) The discovery of the anti-globulin test. *Vox Sanguinis* **45**: 180–3.

National Institute for Clinical Excellence (NICE). (2002) *Guidance on the Use of Routine Antenatal Anti-D Prophylaxis for RhD-Negative Women.* Technology Appraisal 41. London: National Institute for Clinical Excellence.

Nevanlinna H R, Vainio T. (1956) The influence of mother-child ABO incompatibility on Rh immunization. *Vox Sanguinis* **1**: 26–36.

Nijenhuis L E. (1956–7) Blood group frequencies in French Basques. *Acta Genetica et Statistica Medica* **6**: 531–5.

Owen R. (2000) Karl Landsteiner and the first human marker locus. *Genetics* **155**: 995–8.

Pickles M M. (1949) *Haemolytic Disease of the Newborn.* Oxford: Blackwells.

Pickles M M. (1989) The discovery of the enzyme test for Rh antibodies. *Vox Sanguinis* **57**: 223–4.

Pirie N W. (1966) John Burdon Sanderson Haldane. *Biographical Memoirs of Fellows of the Royal Society* **12**: 219–50.

Pollack W, Gorman J G, Freda V J, Ascari W Q, Allen A E, Baker W J. (1968a) Results of clinical trials of RhoGAM in women. *Transfusion* **8**: 151–3.

Pollack W, Gorman J G, Hager H J, Freda V J, Tripode D. (1968b) Antibody-mediated immune suppression to the Rh factor: Animal models suggesting mechanism of action. *Transfusion* **8**: 134–45.

Race R R. (1944) An 'incomplete' antibody in human serum. *Nature* **153**: 771.

Race R R, Sanger R. (1950) *Blood Groups in Man.* 1st edn. Oxford: Blackwell.

Race R R, Sanger R. (1975) *Blood Groups in Man.* 6th edn. Oxford: Blackwell.

Race R R, Sanger R. (1982) Fisher's contribution to Rh. *Vox Sanguinis* **43**: 354–6.

Race R R, Taylor G L, Boorman K E, Dodd B E. (1943) Recognition of Rh genotypes in man. *Nature* **152**: 563–4.

Race R R, Taylor G L, Cappell D F, McFarlane M N. (1944) Recognition of a further Rh genotype in man. *Nature* **153**: 52–3.

Redman T. (1994) Obituaries. Douglas Bevis. *British Medical Journal* **309**: 1013–4.

Robinson A E, Penny A F, Smith J, Tovey D L. (1983) Pilot study for large-scale plasma procurement using automated plasmapheresis. *Vox Sanguinis* **44**: 143–50.

Rodeck C H, Kemp J R, Holman C A, Whitmore D N, Karnicki J, Austin M A. (1981) Direct intravascular fetal blood transfusion by fetoscopy in severe Rhesus isoimmunisation. *Lancet* **i**: 625–7.

Rous P. (1947) Karl Landsteiner 1868–1943. *Obituary Notices of Fellows of the Royal Society* **5**: 295–324.

Schmidt P J. (1994) Rh-Hr: Alexander Wiener's last campaign. *Transfusion* **34**: 180–2.

Singleton B K, Green C A, Avent N D, Martin P G, Smart E, Daka A, Narter-Olaga E, Hawthorne L M, Daniels G. (2000) The presence of an *RhD* pseudogene containing a 37 base pair duplication and a nonsense mutation in Africans with the RhD–negative blood group phenotype. *Blood* **95**: 12–18.

Smith G N, Mollison P L. (1974) Suppression of primary immunisation to the rabbit red cell alloantigen Hg^A by passively administered anti-Hg^A. *Immunology* **26**: 885–92.

Smith T. (1909) Active immunity produced by so-called balanced or neutral mixtures of diphtheria toxin and antitoxin. *Journal of Experimental Medicine* **11**: 241–56.

Soupene E, King N, Field E, Liu P, Niyogi K K, Huang C-H, Kustu S. (2002) Rhesus expression in a green alga is regulated by CO_2. *Proceedings of the National Academy of Sciences* **99**: 7769–73.

Stern K, Goodman H S, Berger M. (1961) Experimental isoimmunization to hemoantigens in man. *Journal of Immunology* **87**: 189–97.

Tansey E M. (1998) 'They used to call it psychiatry': Aspects of the development and impact of psychopharmacology. *Clio Medica* **49**: 79–101.

Tansey E M, Christie D A. (1998) Drugs in psychiatric practice, in Tansey E M, Christie D A, Reynolds L A. (eds) *Wellcome Witnesses to Twentieth Century Medicine*, volume 2. London: The Wellcome Trust, 133–205.

Tansey E M, Christie D A. (1999) Haemophilia: Recent history of clinical management. *Wellcome Witnesses to Twentieth Century Medicine*, volume 4. London: The Wellcome Trust.

Tansey E M, Christie D A. (2000) Looking at the Unborn: Historical aspects of obstetric ultrasound. *Wellcome Witnesses to Twentieth Century Medicine*, volume 5. London: The Wellcome Trust.

Tansey E M, Willhoft S V, Christie D A. (1997) Self and Non-self: A history of autoimmunity, in Tansey E M, Catterall P P, Christie D A, Willhoft S V, Reynolds L A. (eds) *Wellcome Witnesses to Twentieth Century Medicine*, volume 1. London: The Wellcome Trust, 35–66.

Thorpe S J, Sands D, Fox B, Behr-Gross M E, Schäffner G, Yu M W. (2003) Second WHO International Standard for anti-D immunoglobulin. *Vox Sanguinis* **85**: 313–21.

Tovey L A. (1984) The contribution of antenatal anti-D prophylaxis to the reduction of the morbidity and mortality in Rh hemolytic disease of the newborn. *Plasma Therapy Transfusion Technology* **5**: 99–104.

Tovey L A. (1986) Haemolytic disease of the newborn – the changing scene. *British Journal of Obstetrics and Gynaecology* **93**: 960–6.

Tovey L A. (1992) Towards the conquest of Rh haemolytic disease: Britain's contribution and the role of serendipity. Oliver memorial lecture. *Transfusion Medicine* **2**: 99–109.

Tovey L A, Townley A, Stevenson B J, Taverner J. (1983) The Yorkshire antenatal anti-D immunoglobulin trial in primigravidae. *Lancet* **ii**: 244–6.

Urbaniak S J. (1998a) The scientific basis of anti-D prophylaxis. *British Journal of Obstetrics and Gynaecology* **105**: supplement 18, 11–18.

Urbaniak S J. (1998b) Statement from the Consensus Conference on Anti-D Prophylaxis. *Vox Sanguinis* **74**: 127–8.

von Dungern F. (1900) Beiträge zur immunitätslehr. *Munchener Medizinische Wochenschrift* **47**: 677–80.

Walker W, Neligan G A. (1955) Exchange transfusion in haemolytic disease of the newborn. *British Medical Journal* **i**: 681–91.

Walker-Smith J. (2003). *Enduring Memories: A paediatric gastroenterologist remembers, a tale of London and Sydney.* Spennymour: Memoir Club of Whitworth Hall.

Wallerstein H. (1946) Treatment of severe erythroblastosis by simultaneous removal and replacement of blood of the newborn infant. *Science* **103**: 583–4.

Weatherall D. (2002) Sir Cyril Astley Clarke. *Biographical Memoirs of Fellows of the Royal Society* **48**: 69–85.

Wegmann A, Gluck R. (1996) The history of rhesus prophylaxis with anti-D. *European Journal of Pediatrics* **155**: 835–8.

Whitby L E H. (1944) The British Army Blood Transfusion Service. *Journal of the American Medical Association* **124**: 421–4.

Whitfield C. (2000) Rhesus disease: Success but unfinished business. *Year Book of Obstetrics and Gynaecology* **8**: 161–80.

Wiener A S. (1948) Diagnosis and treatment of anemia of the newborn caused by occult placental haemorrhage. *American Journal of Obstetrics and Gynecology* **56**: 717–22.

Wiener A S. (1954) *Rh-Hr Blood Types.* NY: Grune and Stratton.

Wiener A S. (1969) Karl Landsteiner. History of Rh-Hr blood group system. *New York State Journal of Medicine* **69**: 2915–35.

Williamson L M, James V, Duncan S L B, Smith M F. (1989) Plasma exchange for rhesus haemolytic disease: Outcome and follow-up of pregnancies over a 10-year period. *Transfusion Science* **10**: 337–47.

Woodrow J C, Clarke C A, Donohue W T, Finn R, McConnell R B, Sheppard P M, Lehane D, Roberts F M, Gimlette T M. (1975) Mechanism of Rh prophylaxis: An experimental study on specificity of suppression. *British Medical Journal* ii: 57–9.

Yates F, Mather K. (1963) Ronald Aylmer Fisher. *Biographical Memoirs of Fellows of the Royal Society* **9**: 91–130.

Zallen D T. (1999) From butterflies to blood: Human genetics in the United Kingdom, in Fortun M, Mendelsohn E. (eds) *The Practices of Human Genetics.* Dordrecht: Kluwer Academic Publishers, 197–216.

Zallen D T. (2002) The Nuffield Foundation and Medical Genetics in the United Kingdom, in Schneider E W. (ed.) *Rockefeller Philanthropy and Modern Biomedicine.* Bloomington: Indiana University Press.

Zipursky A, Israels LG. (1967) The pathogenesis and prevention of Rh immunization. *Canadian Medical Association Journal.* **97**: 1245–57.

Zipursky A, Hull A, White F D, Israels L G. (1959) Foetal erythrocytes in the maternal circulation. *Lancet* **i**: 451–2.

Zimmerman D R. (1973) *Rh: The Intimate History of a Disease and its Conquest.* New York: Macmillan Publishing Co., Inc.

Biographical notes*

Professor David Anstee
FRCPath FMedSci (b. 1946) has been Director of the International Blood Group Reference Laboratory since 1987 and the Bristol Institute for Transfusion Sciences since 1995. His work has focused on the biochemical characterization of human blood group-active proteins including Rh.

Professor Neil Avent
(b. 1961) is Research Director of the Centre for Research in Biomedicine at University of the West of England (UWE), Bristol, and Co-director of the UWE, Bristol Genomics Research Institute. He was formerly Head of the molecular genetics section (1994–9) at the International Blood Group Reference Laboratory within the National Blood Service, Bristol, which is responsible for the prenatal definition of Rh blood group status in fetuses affected by HDNF. He also was involved in the initial cloning of the Rh protein species (1985–92), which was performed in the Department of Biochemistry, University of Bristol.

Dr Derek Bangham
FRCP (b. 1924) was Head of the Division of Biological Standards at the National Institute for Medical Research (NIMR) from 1961 to 1972, and later Head of the Hormones Division of the National Institute for Biological Standards and Control (NIBSC), from 1972 to 1987.

Dr Barry Benster
FRCOG (b. 1937) trained in Manchester and London and was Rotating Senior Registrar at the Institute of Obstetrics and Gynaecology at Hammersmith Hospital and the Royal University of Malta (1966–71) and then Consultant in Obstetrics and Gynaecology at Huddersfield Royal Infirmary, Huddersfield.

Professor Douglas Bevis
(1919–94) was appointed Senior Lecturer in Obstetrics and Gynaecology at Sheffield University in 1967 and Reader in 1972. He was Professor of Obstetrics and Gynaecology at St James's University Hospital, Leeds, from 1973 until his retirement, working on the use of amniocentesis to determine the prognosis for the fetus in cases of

*Contributors are asked to supply details; others are compiled from conventional biographical sources.

Rh-isoimmunization. See Bevis (1950); Redman (1994).

Dr Frank Boulton
(b. 1941) was Senior Lecturer in Haematology, Liverpool (1975–80), Deputy Director of Edinburgh and South East Scotland Blood Transfusion Service (1980–90), Deputy Director of the Wessex RTC (1990–94) and has been lead Physician, National Blood Service, Southampton, since 1994.

Professor Sir Cyril Clarke
KBE CBE FRCP FRCOG FRS (1907–2000) was Emeritus Professor and Honorary Nuffield Research Fellow in the Department of Genetics at University of Liverpool (1966–76), and established the Nuffield Institute of Medical Genetics there, which he directed from 1963 to 1972. He served as President of the Royal College of Physicians from 1972 to 1977 and received the Lasker Clinical Research Award for work on the genetics of Rh factor, and haemolytic disease of the newborn. See Weatherall (2002).

Professor Robin Coombs
FRS (b. 1921) was Professor of Immunology at the University of Cambridge from 1966 to 1988, then Professor Emeritus. He has been Fellow of Corpus Christi College, Cambridge, since 1962. He developed the antiglobulin test or 'Coombs test', used for the diagnosis of anti-RhD antibodies important in haemolytic disease of the newborn (HDN).

Dr Beryl Corner
FRCP FRCPCH (b. 1910) is Emeritus Consultant Paediatrician, United Bristol Hospitals, and Avon Area Health Authority. She was Clinical Lecturer in Child Health at the University of Bristol from 1937 to 1976. She has consulted for the World Health Organization, in European and South-East Asian regions, particularly for projects in neonatology and child health.

Dr Mahes de Silva
FRCPath (b. 1943) has been lead Consultant for Red Cell Immunohaematology, the National Blood Service, UK, with a major interest in haemolytic disease of the newborn and its prevention.

Dr Sheila Duncan
MD FRCOG (b. 1931) trained in Glasgow and London and was Senior Lecturer/Reader in Obstetrics and Gynaecology at the University of Sheffield from 1969 to 1996. Clinical interests included the management of rhesus-immunized pregnancies during the era of intraperitoneal transfusion in the 1970s and plasmapheresis in the early 1980s. See Williamson *et al.* (1989).

Professor Ronald Finn
FRCP (1930–2004) was Emeritus Consultant Physician, Royal Liverpool University Hospital, and Visiting Professor, Department of Medicine, University of Liverpool. He shared the 1980 Lasker Medical Research Award for his work on the prevention of Rh haemolytic disease. See Freed (2004).

Professor Sir Ronald Fisher
Kt FRS (1890–1962) was Galton Professor of Eugenics at University College London from 1933, and Arthur Balfour Professor of Genetics at the University of Cambridge from 1943 to 1957. See Yates and Mather (1963); Clarke (1990).

Professor Ian Franklin
FRCP FRCPath (b. 1949) was Consultant Haematologist at the Queen Elizabeth Hospital in Birmingham (1982–92), Director of the Bone Marrow Transplant Unit and Consultant Haematologist at the Royal Infirmary, Glasgow (1992–6), Honorary Consultant since 1996, and has been Professor of Transfusion Medicine at the University of Glasgow since 1996 and Medical Director of the Scottish National Blood Transfusion Service (SNBTS) since 1997.

Mr Alistair Gunn
FRCSEd FRCOG (1903–70) was Consulting Obstetrician to the Lewisham and Bromley, Kent, Hospitals and Consulting Gynaecologist to a number of hospitals and public authorities. See Anon. (1971).

Professor John Burdon Sanderson Haldane
FRS (1892–1964) was Professor of Genetics at University College London from 1933 to 1937, and later Professor of Biometry from 1937 to 1957. See Pirie (1966).

Professor Peter Harper
FRCP (b. 1939) is Professor of Medical Genetics at the University of Wales College of Medicine, Cardiff. He has been closely involved with the identification of the genes underlying Huntington's disease and muscular dystrophies, and with their application to predictive genetic testing. He has also been responsible for the development of a general medical service for Wales and has a particular interest in the historical aspects of human and medical genetics. He was awarded a knighthood for services to medicine in 2004. See Harper (1995).

Dr Nevin Hughes-Jones
FRCP FRS (b. 1923) worked in the Medical Research Council's Experimental Haematology (St Mary's Hospital Medical School) and the Molecular Immunopathology Unit (Cambridge) between 1952 and 1988. After retirement, he has continued to work in Cambridge on Rh antigens and their respective antibodies.

Dr Peter Hunter
MRCP (b. 1938) qualified from Middlesex Hospital, London, in 1963 and was Consultant Physician at the Royal Shrewsbury Hospital from 1974 to 1993. From 1994 to 1997 he read pharmacology at King's College London, as preparation for full-time research on the history of discovery of drugs and medicines in the modern era.

Dr Belinda Kumpel
(b. 1948) is a senior research scientist at the Bristol Institute of Transfusion Sciences and the International Blood Group Reference Laboratory which is part of the National Blood Service, sited at Southmead Hospital, Bristol. She made the monoclonal anti-D antibodies that are in clinical development for the prevention of Rh haemolytic disease.

Professor Karl Landsteiner
(1868–1943) is best known for his identification and characterization of the human blood groups, A, B, and O, for which he was awarded the Nobel Prize in Physiology or Medicine in 1930. His research also identified the viral cause of poliomyelitis, also provided the basis for the later development of the polio vaccine. In 1940, with Alexander Wiener, he discovered the Rh factor, which helped to save the lives of many fetuses with mismatched Rh factor from their mothers. See Rous (1947).

Professor Grant Lathe
FCPath (b. 1913) was biochemist at Queen Charlotte's Maternity Hospital, London, from 1949 and Professor of Chemical Pathology, University of Leeds, from 1957 to 1977, now Emeritus.

Dr Philip Levine
(1900–87) was physician and co-discoverer (with Karl Landsteiner and Alexander Wiener) of Rh factors that distinguish different types of human blood cells. See Diamond (1980a); Giblett (1994).

Professor Sir Albert William Liley
Kt FRSNZ FACOG FRCOG (1929–83) did research on neuromuscular transmission before turning to obstetrics at the Women's National Hospital

in Auckland, New Zealand. Liley refined the diagnostic procedure for Rh haemolytic disease of the newborn and was able to predict its severity. In addition, he established the technique of intrauterine transfusion of Rh-negative blood for severely affected fetuses and led the team that carried out the first successful fetal transfusions.

Mr Ian MacKenzie
DSc FRCOG (b. 1942) is Reader in Obstetrics and Gynaecology at the University of Oxford and was the Clinical Director of the Oxford Rhesus Therapy Unit from 1986 to 1996. Along with collaborators he pioneered methods of second-trimester intravascular fetal assessment and transfusion using fetoscopic techniques for treating severe rhesus isoimmunization.

Dr Richard McConnell
FRCP (1920–2003) was a house officer at the David Lewis Northern Hospital, Liverpool, where he met Cyril (later Sir Cyril) Clarke, who was Consultant there at the time. His most important work was in preventing haemolytic disease in newborn babies by administering anti-D serum to Rh-negative women after delivery of a Rh-positive baby. In 1972 they wrote *Prevention of Rhesus Haemolytic Disease.* See Bullamore T. (2004) Richard McConnell. *British Medical Journal* **328**: 111.

Dr Edwin Massey
(b. 1966) has been Consultant Haematologist, National Blood Service and United Bristol Healthcare Trust since 2001.

Professor Patrick Mollison
FRCP FRS (b. 1914) was Director of the MRC Blood Transfusion Research Unit, later Experimental Haematology Unit, from 1946 to 1979 and Professor of Haematology at St Mary's Hospital, London, from 1962 to 1979.

Dr Arthur Ernest Mourant
FRCP FRCPath FRS (1904–94) was Physician, and Director of the Blood Group Reference Laboratory at the Lister Institute. In 1944 he discovered the predicted antibody, anti-E, helping to establish the three-factor theory of the rhesus system. See Misson *et al.* (1999).

Dr Archie Norman
MBE FRCP FRCPI (b. 1912) was Physician to the Hospital for Sick Children, Great Ormond Street, London, from 1950, and Paediatrician to Queen Charlotte's Maternity Hospital, London, from 1952 until his retirement in 1977. From 1976 to 1984 he was Chairman of the Medical Advisory Committee of the Cystic Fibrosis Research Trust.

Mr Elliot Philipp
FRCS FRCOG (b. 1915) was locum Consultant Obstetrician at Lewisham Hospital (1952), Consultant Obstetrician and Gynaecologist at Old Church Hospital, Romford (1952–64) and Consultant in Obstetrics and Gynaecology at the Royal Northern, City of London, and Whittington Hospitals (1964–80).

Dr Robert Race
CBE FRS (1907–84) was Director of the Medical Research Council Blood Group Unit from 1946 to 1973. See Clarke (1985).

Dr Angela Robinson
FRCPath (b. 1942) has been Medical Director of the National Blood Service since 1995, Director of the Yorkshire Blood Transfusion Service (1989–95) and Consultant Paediatric Haematologist, transfusion medicine specialist and Senior Lecturer at the University of Leeds from 1976 to 1989.

Professor Charles Rodeck
FRCOG FRCPath FMedSci (b. 1944) is Professor of Obstetrics and Gynaecology and Head of Department at University College London, and Director of the Fetal Medicine Unit at University College London Hospitals. His research and clinical practice have been in prenatal diagnosis and the emerging discipline of fetal medicine. He established the first fetal medicine unit in the UK, the Harris Birthright Centre at King's College Hospital, in 1983, and further departments of fetal medicine at Queen Charlotte's Maternity Hospital (1986), and University College Hospital (1990). He has been President of the International Society for Prenatal Diagnosis since 2002.

Dr Ruth Sanger
FRS (1918–2001) was on the Scientific Staff of the Medical Research Council Blood Group Unit from 1946 to 1983, and Director of the Unit from 1973 to 1983. See Mollison (2002); Hughes-Jones and Tippett (2003).

Professor James Scott
FRCSEd FRCOG (b. 1924) was Professor of Obstetrics and Gynaecology (1961–89), and Dean of the Faculty of Medicine (1986–9), University of Leeds, having trained in Scotland, Ireland and elsewhere in England. He was a Wellcome Research Fellow at Northwestern University, Chicago and has been Visiting Professor in other centres in the USA, Australia and New Zealand.

Professor Philip Sheppard
HonFRCP FRS (1921–76) was Professor of Genetics at the University of Liverpool, from 1963 and his research on rhesus blood groups led to the method of preventing rhesus haemolytic disease of the newborn. He was awarded the Darwin Medal of the Royal Society in 1974 and the Gold Medal of the Linnean Society in 1975. See Clarke (1977).

Dr John Silver
FRCP (b. 1931) was Consultant-in-Charge of the Liverpool Regional Paraplegic Centre (1965–70) and Consultant in Spinal Injuries at the National Spinal Injuries Centre, Stoke Mandeville Hospital, Aylesbury, Bucks, from 1970 until 1992. Since his retirement he has been engaged in research work on spinal injuries and medical history.

Dr Jean Smellie
FRCP HonFRCPCH (b. 1927) qualified at Oxford and then University College Hospital, London, in 1950. She trained in paediatrics at the Royal Manchester Children's Hospital, Great Ormond Street, University College Hospital and Oxford, between 1952 and 1961. She was Honorary Consultant Paediatrician and Senior Lecturer, University College Hospital, London, from 1970 to 1993, later Emeritus, and Honorary Consultant Paediatric Nephrologist at Guy's and Great Ormond Street Hospitals, Honorary Senior Lecturer in Community Child Health, Southampton, from 1984 to 1992.

Dr Patricia Tippett
(b. 1930) was a member of the Medical Research Council Blood Group Unit from 1958 to 1995 and became Director of the Unit when Ruth Sanger retired in 1983.

Dr Derrick Tovey
FRCPath FRCOG (b. 1926) was Director of the Yorkshire Region Transfusion Centre (1966–88) and Chairman of the Anti-D Working Party, Department of Health and Social Security (~1980–88).

Dr Geoffrey Harold Tovey
CBE FRCP FRCPath (1916–2001) became a lecturer in haematology at Bristol University (1948), Founder and Director of the UK Transplant Service and President of the International Society of Blood Transfusion (1972), President of the British Society for Haematology (1977) and in 1978 became Consultant Advisor to the Department of Health. See Fraser (2002).

Professor Timos Valaes
(b. 1927) after graduating from the Medical School in Athens he obtained his paediatric training in England and an MD from Bristol University. He became Director of the Institute of Child Health in Athens. He moved to Boston in 1974 and became Chief of the Neonatology service of the New England Medical Center, Boston, and Professor of Paediatrics (Emeritus since 2000) at Tufts University School of Medicine.

Professor William Walker
FRCP FRCPath (1919–98) was a pioneer in the treatment of rhesus haemolytic disease of the newborn and became an expert in the technique of exchange transfusion. See Craft (2004).

Mr Humphry Ward
FRCOG (b. 1938) undertook initial training in Auckland, NZ, with Professor William (later Sir William) Liley. He was a Consultant Obstetrician and Gynaecologist and Senior Clinical Lecturer at University College Hospital and University College Hospital Medical School, London (1972–2000), until retirement.

Professor Sir David Weatherall
Kt FRCP FRCPE FRS (b. 1933) was Professor of Haematology at the University of Liverpool from 1971 to 1974, and Nuffield Professor of Clinical Medicine at the University of Oxford from 1974 to 1992. From 1992 to 2000 he was Regius Professor of Medicine at the University of Oxford; and Honorary Director of the Molecular Haematology Unit of the Medical Research Council from 1980 to 2000 and the Institute for Molecular Medicine from 1988 to 2000 (renamed the Weatherall Institute of Molecular Medicine from 2000).

Sir Lionel Whitby
MC Kt CVO FRCP (1895–1956) was Regius Professor of Physic at Cambridge University from 1945 until his death. He headed the Army Blood Transfusion Service from 1939 to 1945. His research at the Bland Sutton Institute, London, focused on pathology, bacteriology and haematology, and included collaborative work that led to the development and successful production of sulphapyridine (M&B693). See Whitby and Dodds (1931); Anon. (1957, 1968).

Professor Charles Whitfield
FRCOG (b. 1927) was Consultant Obstetrician and Honorary Reader in Belfast (to 1974), Professor of Obstetrics, University of Manchester (1974–6) and Regius

Professor of Midwifery, University of Glasgow (1976–92). He established the tertiary referral services for Rh disease in Northern Ireland and at The Queen Mother's Hospital, Glasgow. He is a member of the Joint Subcommittee on Prevention of Haemolytic Disease of the Newborn. See Whitfield (2000).

Dr Alexander Wiener
FACP (1907–76) was Senior Serologist to the Office of the Chief Medical Examiner of NY City and Head of the Transfusion Division, The Jewish Hospital of Brooklyn, NY. Much of his work is described in Wiener (1954). See also Moor-Jankowski (1978); Schmidt (1994).

Professor John Woodrow
FRCP (b. 1924) was on the staff of the Department of Medicine at the University of Liverpool between 1961 and 1991, and was Consultant Physician (General Medicine and Rheumatology) to the Liverpool United Hospitals.

Professor Doris Zallen
(b. 1941) is Professor of Science and Technology Studies at Virginia Polytechnic Institute and State University in Blacksburg, Virginia. A former laboratory scientist who has made contributions to cell biology and linkage testing, she now conducts research on the history of genetics and on the ethical, social and policy issues related to genetic testing and other clinical uses of genetics.

Glossary

Bold text within a definition indicates another glossary entry.

Afibrinogenaemia
A rare disease where the blood has difficulty clotting due to the lack of fibrinogen, or clotting factor I.

Amniocentesis
A procedure in which a needle is passed transabdominally into the amniotic sac to obtain a sample of amniotic fluid. The optical density of the fluid is measured to give an assessment of the degree of fetal haemolysis (the rate of red blood cell destruction, caused by the rhesus antibodies).

Amniotic fluid
The fluid surrounding the developing fetus, found within the amniotic sac contained in the mother's uterus.

Bilirubin
The orange-yellow pigment of bile, the fluid that aids digestion and is secreted by the liver.

Contig
A set of overlapping segments of DNA.

Disseminated intravascular coagulation (DIC)
Intravascular coagulation where many coagulation factors are depleted. It can be induced by different factors including infection in the blood by bacteria or fungus, severe tissue injury as in burns and head injury, cancer, reactions to blood transfusions, and obstetrical complications such as retained placenta after delivery. See also **afibrinogenaemia.**

Erythroblastosis fetalis
Severe anaemia in newborn babies; the result of Rh incompatibility between maternal and fetal blood which typically occurs when the child of an Rh-negative mother inherits Rh-positive blood from the father. This can be diagnosed before birth by **amniocentesis.**

Friedreich ataxia
A hereditary disease in which there is degeneration of the nerves in the spinal cord, the cerebellum and of sensory nerves to the hands and feet. It starts in childhood or adolescence, marked by an unsteady gait and an inability to coordinate voluntary movements.

Haemolytic disease of newborn (HDN) (rhesus disease)
The condition caused by Rh-positive cells from a fetus with a Rh-positive father finding their way into the circulation of a Rh-negative mother, usually at birth, and inducing antibody formation

to what is, for her, a foreign antigen. In the next pregnancy her antibodies are transferred to the fetus across the placenta (a normal protective process) and attack the baby's red blood cells if they are Rh positive, inducing haemolysis and causing anaemia and **jaundice.** This sequence of events can be prevented by giving women antibodies to Rh-positive cells at delivery, thus preventing her sensitization. Some cases of haemolytic disease result from maternal transfer of naturally occurring antibody to her fetus, such as may occur with an A or B group fetus and an O group mother. See also **kernicterus**.

Hydrops fetalis

Oedema of the entire body due to abnormal accumulation of serous fluid in the tissues, associated with severe anaemia and occurring in fetal **erythroblastosis.**

Kernicterus

Kernicterus may occur when there is a high level of unconjugated **bilirubin** in the circulating blood such as in **haemolytic disease of the newborn**, but much more commonly in **premature** babies who tend to have a deficiency of liver enzymes for conjugation of **bilirubin**. High levels of unconjugated **bilirubin** can pass the immature blood-brain barrier of the newborn and cause degeneration of cells of the basal ganglia and hippocampus resulting in seizure, cerebral palsy and in severe cases death.

Jaundice

A condition caused by obstruction of the bile and accumulation of bile pigment (**bilirubin**) and characterized by yellowing of the skin and whites of the eyes.

Peritoneum

A transparent membrane that lines the abdominal cavity in mammals and covers most of the viscera.

Petechiae

Pinpoint-sized haemorrhages of small capillaries in the skin or mucous membranes.

Plasmapheresis

The procedure whereby plasma is removed, separated and extracted from anticoagulated whole blood and the remaining red blood cells are returned to the patient.

Preterm (premature) birth

The birth of a baby before 37 weeks of gestation (calculated from the first day of the mother's last menstrual period). Very preterm is birth before 33 weeks.

Rhesus (Rh) factor

A blood protein that may cause severe complications in pregnancy.

People without Rh factor are known as Rh negative (or RhD negative), while people with the Rh factor are Rh positive (or RhD positive). If a woman who is Rh negative is pregnant with a fetus that is Rh positive, her body may make antibodies against the fetus's blood. This can cause Rh disease, also known as **haemolytic disease of the newborn**, in the baby.

Sagittal sinus
A large vein that goes over the top of the skull from front to back and then splits to take blood from the brain back toward the heart.

Thrombocytopaenia
A deficiency of platelets often associated with haemorrhage.

Trimester
A period of three months. During pregnancy, the first trimester continues until week 13, the second trimester from week 13 to 28, and the third trimester from week 28 until delivery.

Index: Subject

Index: Names

Biographical notes appear in bold

Key to photographs

Front cover, top to bottom

Professor Sir David Weatherall

Professor John Woodrow

Professor Ronald Finn*

Professor Doris Zallen

This page, top to bottom

Dr Sheila Duncan

Mr Elliot Philipp

Dr Nevin Hughes-Jones

Professor Ian Franklin

*Died 21 May 2004

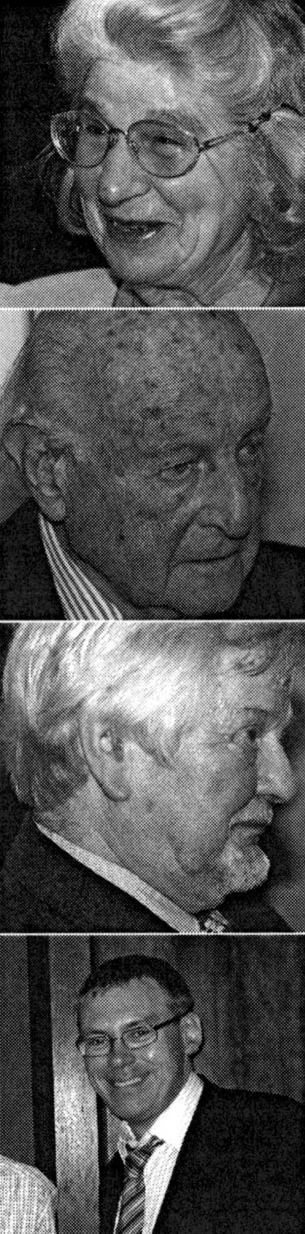

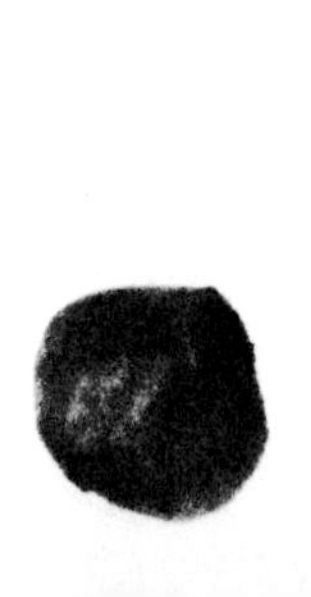

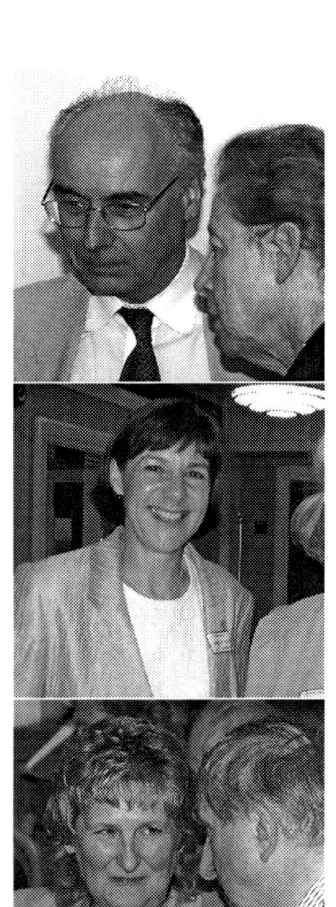

Key to photographs

Back cover, top to bottom
Professor Patrick Mollison
Professor Robin Coombs
Dr Beryl Corner
Dr Derrick Tovey

This page, top to bottom
Professor Charles Rodeck
Dr Belinda Kumpel
Dr Angela Robinson
Professor Charles Whitfield

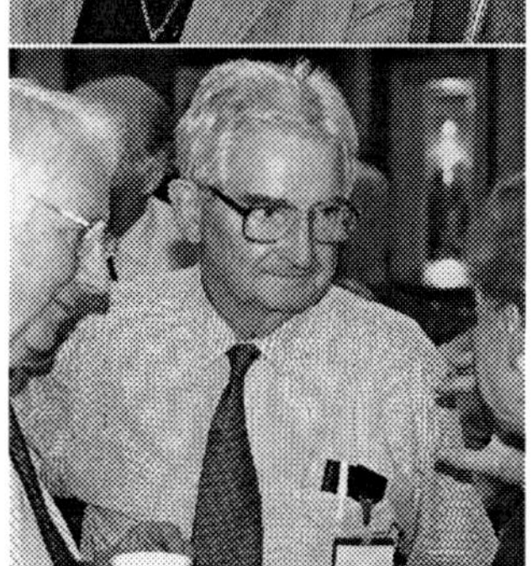

CPSIA information can be obtained at www.ICGtesting.com
Printed in the USA
LVOW051503290512

283769LV00007B/8/A

9 780854 840991